$12.95

TENTH EDITION

A NATURAL METHOD OF HEALTH CARE

Introduction To Chiropractic

By Louis Sportelli, D.C.

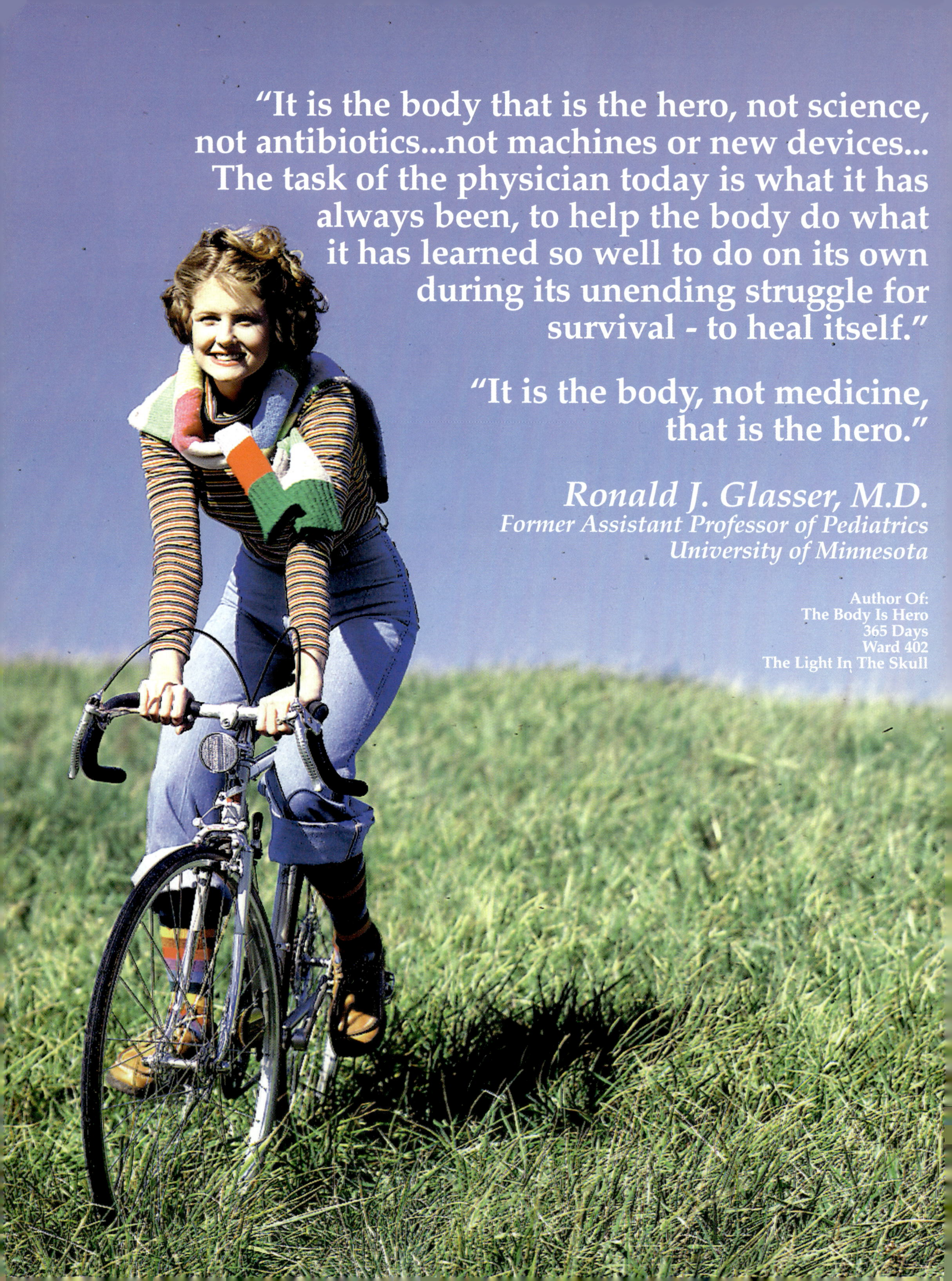

"It is the body that is the hero, not science, not antibiotics...not machines or new devices... The task of the physician today is what it has always been, to help the body do what it has learned so well to do on its own during its unending struggle for survival - to heal itself."

"It is the body, not medicine, that is the hero."

Ronald J. Glasser, M.D.
Former Assistant Professor of Pediatrics
University of Minnesota

Author Of:
The Body Is Hero
365 Days
Ward 402
The Light In The Skull

Table Of Contents

Facts You Should Know About Chiropractic

- Chiropractic was established in 1895.
- Chiropractic is the second largest of the three primary health care professions in the United States and growing each year.
- There are approximately 65,000 doctors of chiropractic in the United States and another 20,000 around the world. According to recent surveys, there has been a significant increase in the utilization of chiropractic health care by the general population. The growth pattern indicates that the figures will increase substantially in the next decade.
- All 50 states, Puerto Rico, the District of Columbia, and the U.S. Virgin Islands have statutes recognizing and regulating the practice of chiropractic as an independent health service.
- Board-qualified and licensed chiropractors are entitled by law to use the title “Doctor of Chiropractic,” “D.C.” and/or “Chiropractic Physician”.
- Chiropractic health care is provided for in such federal programs as Medicare, the Government Employees Hospital Association Benefit Plan, The Mailhandlers Benefit Plan, and the Postmasters Benefit Plan.
- State Medicaid Acts in most states include doctors of chiropractic as primary health providers.
- Chiropractic benefits are provided for in health insurance policies of virtually every major insurance carrier, State Workers’ Compensation Program, and the Federal Employee's Compensation Act (FECA). A substantial number of major international, national and local labor unions provide chiropractic services in their health and welfare plans, as do many major industrial employers. A high percentage of managed care organizations in the United States, estimated at 75%, cover chiropractic services. The various managed care plans have a wide range of coverage benefits depending on the employer, insurance company, union contract or particular health care benefit plan.
- All Federal agencies accept sick-leave certificates signed by doctors of chiropractic, and fees paid to doctors of chiropractic are allowable deductions as expenses for “medical care” for Federal income tax purposes.
- The typical doctor of chiropractic’s training includes an eight-year program of undergraduate and professional college study and clinic internship prior to entering private practice. The areas of science studied are those pertinent to the health care of human beings, including diagnosis, anatomy, bacteriology, pathology, physiology, biochemistry, pediatrics, geriatrics, spinal manipulation, x-ray, nutrition, physical therapeutics and many other appropriate subjects.
- The professional accrediting agency for chiropractic colleges is the Commission on Accreditation of the Council on Chiropractic Education (CCE). The Accrediting Commission of the CCE is recognized by the U.S. Department of Education and the Council for Higher Education Accreditation (CHEA). It is included in the Department’s list of nationally recognized accrediting agencies and associations.
- The G.I. Bill of Rights covers education in chiropractic colleges for qualified veterans.
- Wide acceptance and a rapidly increasing population make the future of chiropractic optimistic. There is a changing model of health care emerging from a disease model to a wellness model. Chiropractic is a non-drug and non-surgical health profession. Career opportunities are plentiful for young men and women desiring to enter chiropractic.
- The chiropractic profession adheres to a standard of ethics. Members of national professional associations, as well as state associations, are provided with a code of ethics. The public should expect and demand high professional standards.
- To find out more information about chiropractic, we suggest you use the website: www.chiroweb.com/find/firstvisit.html

Introduction

From Hippocrates (The Father of Medicine) and Galen (The Prince of Physicians) to the 19th-century bonesetters of the British Isles, many individuals throughout history have recognized the importance of the spine and nervous system as they relate to the health of the individual. The wisdom of this concept is even more compelling as our society becomes more dependent on drugs or surgery for treatment of health problems. However, in the broad tapestry of health care, the golden thread of manipulation weaves its way throughout.

The author does not wish to imply that there is never a sound need for drugs or surgery. To advocate such would be provincial and unrealistic in light of the sophistication of science and technology.

However, with increased knowledge has also come a greater appreciation for natural, conservative methods as viable alternatives for many human ailments. This booklet attempts to provide insight into the "holistic" (total person) concept of health care, which the chiropractic profession has long championed. Doctors of chiropractic have been recognized as providing exceptional care for back pain, headaches and other spinal related disorders. A fact many people have not known is that doctors of chiropractic have been proponents of the capacity and integrity of the body and mind to deal with stress and disease, and have criticized the overuse and abuse of drugs and unnecessary surgery. Evidence today suggests that "watchful waiting" as a preliminary management plan may avoid unnecessary treatment.

Chiropractic care, seeks to restore normal physiologic function and thereby help to improve the health of the individual. Counseling patients in areas such as nutrition, proper exercise and diet, lifestyle changes and general health matters demonstrates the doctor of chiropractic's concern about the "whole person." Chiropractic adjustments attempt to restore proper spinal motion, and thereby directly influences spinal-related disorders. Some authorities suggest that adjustments to the spine also have the potential to influence neural integrity and thus affect dysfunction of internal organs.

For more than a century, doctors of chiropractic have advocated that an optimally functioning nervous system is necessary to good health. The significance of the nervous system, and its influence on the body's ability to adapt to its environment, is becoming more and more relevant as research continues to advance, seeking the answers to how the body is able to respond and activate its immune system to protect the whole person.

As society moves into the 21st century, there is increased awareness of the need to consider prevention and health maintenance rather than simply waiting for a disease to be found and treated. What may initially have been considered an alternative approach to health care has now become mainstream for tens of millions of Americans who seek better health and increased personal participation in the way their care is provided.

Hopefully, this booklet will serve to provide a basic understanding of the science, art, and philosophy of chiropractic.

Louis Sportelli, D.C.

What Is Chiropractic?

Perhaps this book is your first introduction to chiropractic as a health care profession. If this is the case, you probably have some questions pertaining to what chiropractic is, and how the natural conservative approach of chiropractic may aid in relieving many health ailments. Most people know chiropractic care is outstanding in the treatment of back pain, neck pain and headaches. Many do not know about chiropractic, and how it can help many other health ailments. Hopefully this booklet will provide a much clearer understanding about the chiropractic profession.

If, on the other hand, you are familiar with chiropractic, this booklet will serve as a gentle refresher about the profession.

What is chiropractic? What does a chiropractor do? Is there a way I can improve my health without drugs? How long will I take to note improvement? Can chiropractic help children? Are exercise and lifestyle important to my health? Can senior citizens benefit from chiropractic care? Do I need to be x-rayed?

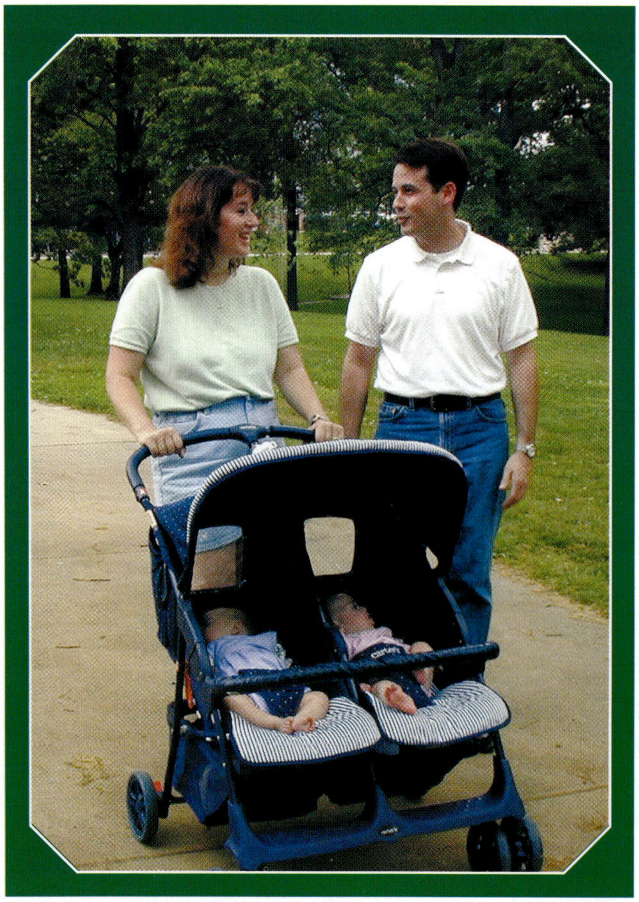

These and many more questions will be answered. We will attempt to explain the conservative, "drugless" approach your doctor of chiropractic utilizes in aiding you to become a happier, healthier person who enjoys a sense of well-being.

Chiropractic is a branch of the healing arts, and as a health-care discipline is based on the premise that good health depends, in part, upon a normally functioning nervous system. When body structures such as cells and organs are functioning normally, a state of health or normal physiology exists. However, when the body's physiology is abnormal the potential for a disease state exists. Thus, we begin to understand that abnormal physiology and function predispose the body to disease processes.[1,2,3,4,5]

The spinal cord has 31 pairs of spinal nerves which exit from the spinal column (backbone). The most delicate and important organs of the nervous system (brain and spinal cord) are encased in hard bony coverings composed of the skull and spinal vertebrae. The spine provides protection, mobility, and weight bearing support for our upright position. The spine offers protection to the delicate spinal nerves which exit from the spinal column. Irritation to the spinal nerves can occur when spinal bio-mechanics are compromised and not functioning properly.

Chiropractors have maintained the body possesses well-designed "survival mechanisms" intended to maintain the body in a state of good health. The body's ability to cope goes far beyond the widely known "fight or flight" responses to stress-

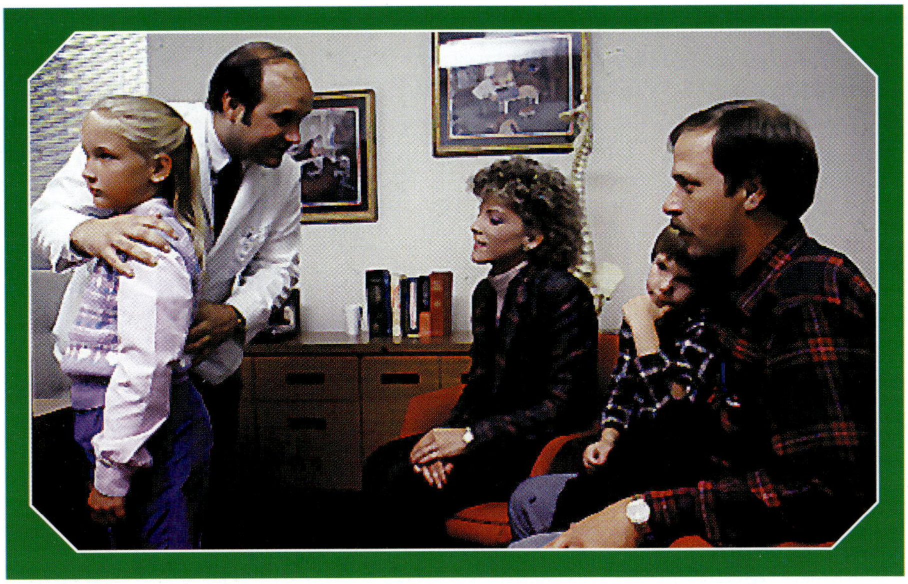

A Natural Method Of Health Care

ful situations. These additional mechanisms might have a great deal to do with the psychological "stressors" and how an individual responds to stress and its influence on the individual's predisposition to disease. These concepts were described in early chiropractic writings which discussed the body's "innate intelligence" over 100 years ago.[6,7,8] Now more and more authorities are discussing these issues in contemporary publications on wellness.[9] The link between mind and body is one of the basic tenets of the newly developing science of psychoneuro-immunology[10,11] and which has been part of the foundation of chiropractic theory.

Do you have to tell your body to digest the food you eat? Do you have to tell your heart how many times to beat? Do you tell your lungs when to breathe? Do you have to direct your body to heal and repair a cut finger? Do you have to order your immune system to overcome an outbreak of flu or an infection? You see, the body has the ability to function and *keep you well*, provided it is not compromised. Doctors of chiropractic do not utilize drugs or surgery in their practices. They believe that the body responds to stressful conditions in a more organized and specific manner than generalized "fight or flight" responses.[12] There is also close communication between the central nervous system, the immune system, and hormones as well — as suggested in figure 1, page 12.[13] Chiropractic strategies of health management recognize and seek to optimize these interactions and traditionally have approached the spine and nervous system as key elements in maintaining overall health. If other methods of treatment are indicated, however, your doctor of chiropractic will recommend that you consult with a medical or other health care practitioner for specific treatment you may require.

Chiropractic Concepts Of Health Maintenance

Throughout history, man has been searching for that mythical *"Fountain of Youth."* This quest for eternal youth and well-being effects the health care industry. Billions of dollars are spent annually on elixirs, fad diets, rejuvenation resorts, cosmetic surgery and the like. Countless hours and much effort are being spent to look "young and healthy." But do many achieve that goal?

What is this thing called "health?" It is more than just the absence of disease. Health must be viewed as an evolving state, a process that starts at birth and continues until death. The health care crisis now raging throughout our country has caused many people to start asking some very pointed questions about the type of care they are receiving and whether the current model of health care needs to be changed. Terms that appear in almost all discussions relating to health care are, *"maintenance,"* and *"disease prevention."*

The concept of health maintenance is not new to the chiropractic profession. Throughout chiropractic's more than 100-year history, its practitioners have promoted the concept of the body's ability to adapt to its environment: Thus the need to maintain the nervous system free from neurological irritation. Many chiropractors hold as a basic tenet that many disease processes involve an improperly functioning nerve supply to the body organs or tissues. Chiropractic health care primarily focuses on examining and evaluating the spine and pelvis to determine if any one area of the spine is malfunctioning or if many areas of the spine are causing abnormal body movements. If present, these subluxations (malfunctions) may contribute to stresses that influence the nervous system and compromise its ability to adapt and function.

We have been taught since childhood that if there are *"no symptoms,"* we are well. We have been preconditioned by advertising media to believe that anytime a symptom appears we need simply "pop this pill" or "swallow that liquid," and all will be well. Drugs and medications have become so commonplace that we do not question whether we should take them or not, but rather, which ones are "faster" or "stronger."

In reality, we often only hide the problem (symptom) by medicating it. We do many things to fool ourselves into thinking we are well: avoiding activities which cause pain; not eating foods which cause distress; by attributing suggestions to "just getting older." By continuing to approach our health in this fashion, we are in essence avoiding or masking the symptoms, rather than attempting to identify the underlying cause of the body's malfunction.

This approach makes as much sense as building hospitals to treat accident victims rather than installing traffic lights to prevent accidents.

The chiropractic approach to well-being typifies the new and changing attitude toward health. It is based on the concept of "maintaining health" versus "treating disease."

When a person understands the chiropractic concept of health maintenance, advertising gimmicks, catchy phrases and clever jingles lose their attraction. The premise that the body (unless it has a genetic [inborn] deficiency) is capable of maintaining health, when given proper, essential ingredients is basic to chiropractic. Adequate nutrition, water, rest, clean air, exercise and a properly functioning nervous system, as well as a positive attitude, are critical requirements for maintenance of good health.

Chiropractic health maintenance is gaining in acceptance and public support because its concepts and ideas about health care are well-founded and rational. For example, the chiropractic profession has frequently spoken out on health issues such as the overuse and abuse of drugs, tobacco and alcohol, the increasing rate of iatrogenic (doctor caused) diseases and many other environmental and social issues which affect the quality of our lives.

Chiropractors teach that health is not a commodity which can be purchased in a tablet or bottle; it can only be obtained and maintained by allowing the natural recuperative powers of the body to function unimpaired. Locating and correcting spinal subluxations (deviations) early may help to prevent more serious conditions from developing.[14]

Today, we read about "health maintenance" as if it were some new and revolutionary discovery. Health maintenance is being emphasized by every group interested in the delivery of health care. Chiropractic has for many years offered a stimulating challenge to people interested in an alternative to the usual "treat only the symptom" type of care.

A few simple questions can help determine the type of health care best suited to each individual's needs.

"Why did I get sick?" "Is it because some mysterious virus or germ singled me out to be sick?" "Am I sick because my body has a low resistance which allowed me to become susceptible to a disease process?" "What is the cause of the problem?"

These questions can be better understood by dealing with the underlying problem, rather than masking the symptoms on a temporary basis, which often allows the illness to become more serious. The benefits of this health maintenance approach are becoming more obvious every day. The chiropractic profession teaches the advantages of looking at the individual as a whole person (holistic) rather than treating the effects of an isolated symptom.

Health maintenance is gaining considerable support by those who understand the significance of this concept. Health cannot be purchased in a bottle, substituted or stored, but it can be lost very quickly. If health could be purchased with money, we would have no sick millionaires.

In this booklet, we will explain and illustrate the concept of chiropractic as a health profession. Your doctor of chiropractic (D.C.) may suggest when you should return so he can monitor your condition and determine the need for care. The interval and procedure will be tailored to your individual needs and health problems. Characteristics such as weight, lifestyle, stress (emotional and physical), occupation, age, spinal abnormalities, and details in your personal health profile, will be considered by your doctor when he or she makes a determination about your case.

Many people find that regular chiropractic care, as part of a total healthcare program, enables them to function and perform to a higher potential. Outcome measures are continually being developed to determine the effectiveness of chiropractic healthcare.[15,16] A preliminary report from Alternative Medicine, Inc. (AMI), which is a multi-specialty group, promoted the use of doctors of chiropractic as primary care providers. The data, while preliminary, suggests that using chiropractors as the entry provider reduced global health care costs by more than 50 percent. Further analysis of this data will occur in 2000 and 2001.[95] The public is becoming more aware of the benefits of this approach to health. Millions of people are now utilizing chiropractic services for their health care needs.

What Does A Doctor Of Chiropractic (D.C.) Do?

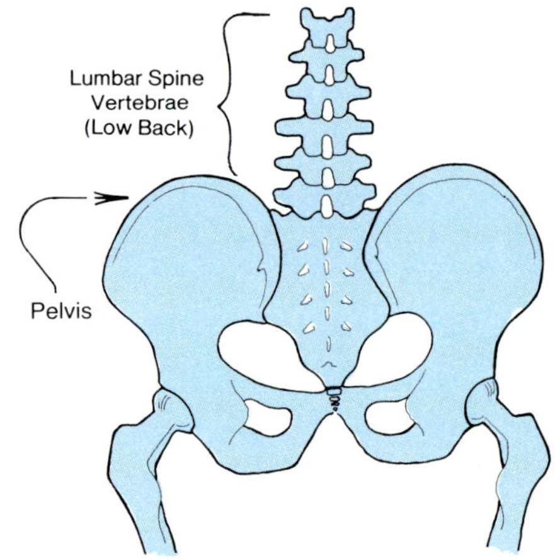

Lower Spine & Pelvis
Viewed from the rear

Most doctors use a standard procedure of examination to diagnose a patient's condition. Your doctor of chiropractic uses time honored methods of consultation, case history, physical examination, and when indicated, X-rays or other modern imaging tests or laboratory analysis to arrive at a diagnosis. In addition, he or she provides a careful chiropractic structural examination, with special emphasis on the spine, extremities,nervous and musculoskeletal system.

The examination of your spine and muscle system to evaluate structure and function is what makes the chiropractic approach different from that of other health care practitioners.

Your spinal column, or vertebral column, is a series of movable bones which begin at the base of your skull and end at your hips. Although the spine is composed of 24 individual vertebrae, it functions as one dynamic structure upon which the total body skeleton is dependent for support and movement. There are seven cervical (neck) vertebrae, twelve dorsal (mid-back) vertebrae, and five lumbar (low-back) vertebrae. These vertebrae are stacked up like building blocks, with discs (shock absorbers) between them. These discs help to cushion shock, reduce friction, bind the vertebrae together, and allow movement to occur more easily.

Thirty-one pair of spinal nerves extend down the spine from the brain and exit through a series of openings between the vertebrae. The nerves leave the spine and form a very complicated network which ultimately influences every living tissue in your body.

Accidents, falls, uneven stress, tension, over-exertion or other factors may not allow the spine to move properly within its normal range of motion. This can result in minor displacements or derangements of one or more of these vertebrae, causing irritation to spinal nerve roots directly by pressure or indirectly through reflexes.

These irritations, in turn, may cause malfunctions in your body. Many chiropractors believe that nerve pressure, or nerve reflex changes, can cause a disturbance to delicate body functions resulting in an increased susceptibility to disease processes. Spinal subluxations (lesions) have been shown to cause improper function of organs, leading to increased susceptibility to infection or chronic disease.[8,17,18]

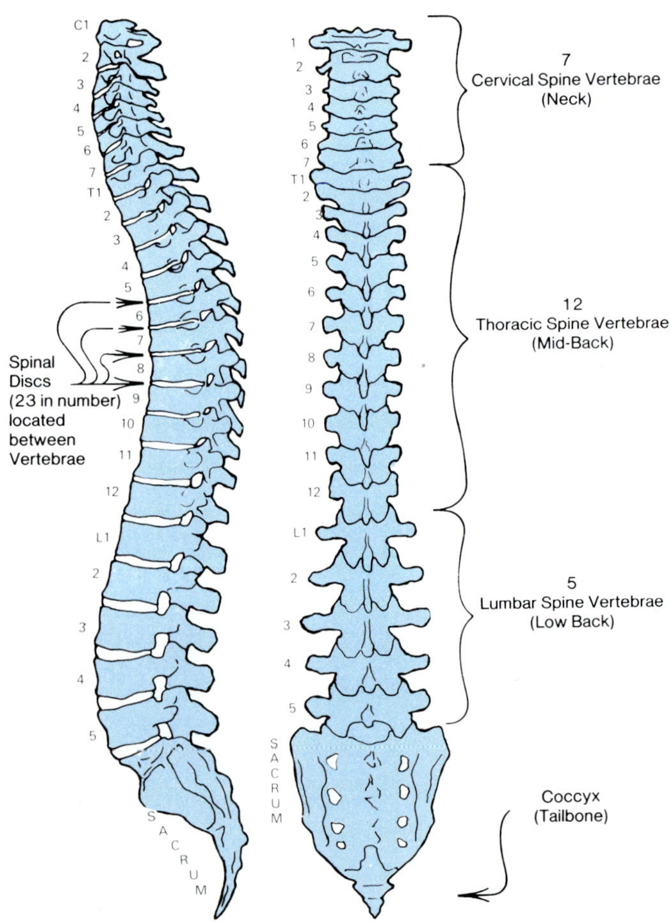

Viewed from left side

Viewed from the rear

Facts About The Nervous System

The following three illustrations show the different parts of the total nervous system. They are shown in the three main divisions, on the basis of anatomy and specific functions. While the breakdown is used for illustration purposes, each segment of the nervous system is interdependent and interrelated. The body is so wonderfully complex that one part often affects another part seemingly distant, remote, and unrelated.[3,19] Therefore, the spine is the doctor of chiropractic's "avenue of approach." The doctor will attempt to influence malfunctioning parts of the body through a careful examination and subsequent manipulations (adjustments) of the offending spinal vertebrae and/or other structural lesions which may be present.

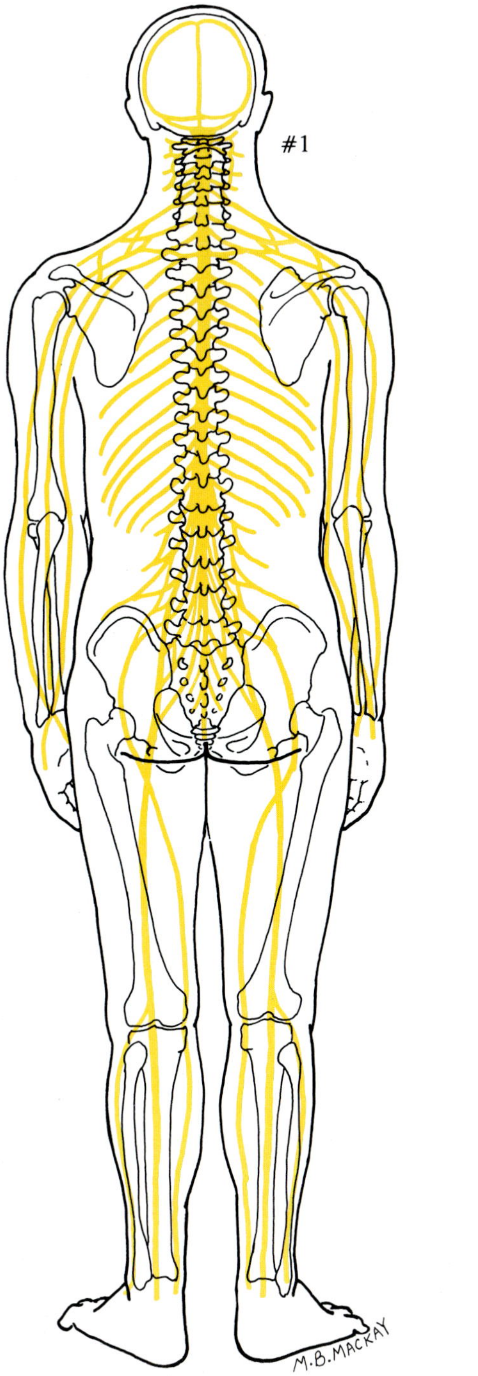

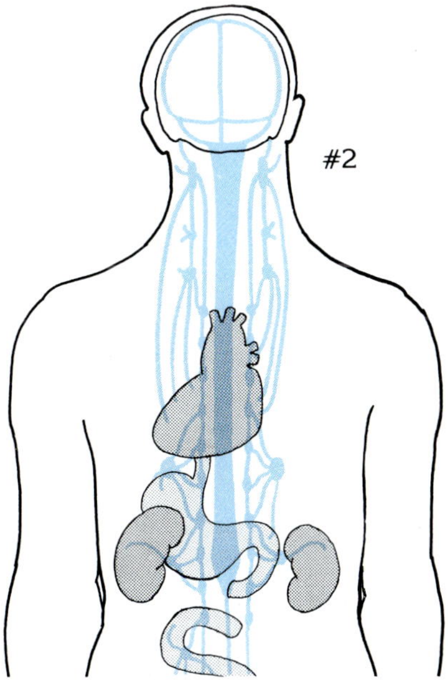

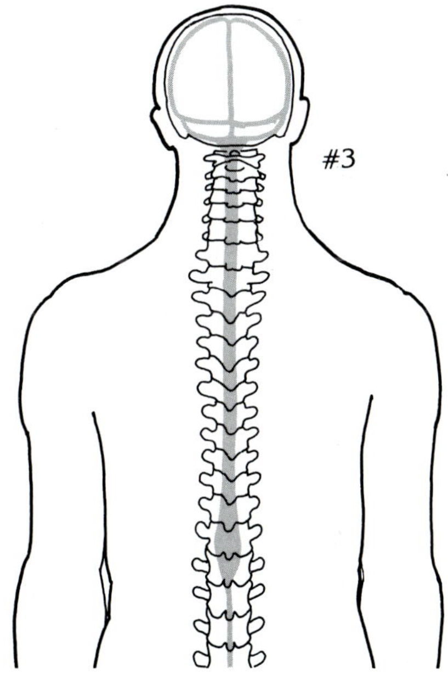

#1 The Peripheral Nervous System serves to connect the central nervous system with the various tissues of the body. Spinal nerves at various levels have sensory and motor connections. Messages or signals can be relayed from the tissues of the body back to the brain through the spinal cord. The spinal nerves extend outward from the spinal cord through openings between the vertebrae. Once they pass through these openings, they extend great distances dividing into many branches, thus forming a complicated, intricate network reaching all the tissues of the body. The peripheral nervous system is composed of Cranial nerves, Spinal nerves, and the Autonomic nervous system.

#2 The Autonomic Nervous System, or "involuntary nervous system," as it is sometimes called, governs those activities which are carried out automatically without the individual being conscious of their performance. Examples of these activities would be regulation of heartbeat, digestion of food, circulation of blood, etc. It has two divisions, the "Sympathetic" and "Parasympathetic" which in general serve to produce opposite and equalizing effects on the body to maintain it in a state of "balance."

#3 The Central Nervous System, includes the brain and spinal cord. The brain is encased in a hard protective covering: the skull. The spinal cord is encased in the center of the spinal vertebrae for protection. The functions of the body are truly examples of engineering marvels not to be duplicated or yet to be fully understood.

What Kinds Of Conditions Do Chiropractors Treat?

When chiropractic was first introduced to the world in 1896, it represented a new and different approach to the problems of healthcare. At that time, the approach was centered upon specific diseases, such as gastritis, headaches, ulcers, colitis and other disorders. People tended to think of a specific treatment for each known disease.

One common method for the treatment of disease consists primarily of putting chemicals or drugs into the body in an attempt to bring the body back to health. On the other hand, the chiropractic profession, with its natural, drugless approach to health, maintains that the body ordinarily receives all the nutrients it needs to achieve good health through the proper balance of food, oxygen and water consumed by eating, drinking and breathing. Chiropractors suggest that when disease occurs, one cause is often related to the body's failing to digest, absorb, or metabolize food appropriately or to properly eliminate wastes from the body.

Chiropractic has given the world a different and drugless concept of health, stressing the fact that many disease processes begin with the body's inability to adapt to its environment. Chiropractic's approach to treating human ills was not to look for the cure in drugs or chemicals, but to locate an area that was deficient in nerve supply, nutrition or circulation. Without unfettered nerve supply the body is not able to perform to its full potential. If chiropractic had not embraced a different approach to health care, the profession would not have continued to expand and flourish into one of the largest drugless healthcare professions in the world. The unique benefit of chiropractic's clinical approach has restored good health to millions of people, often after other methods have failed. There may be times, however, when your body is not able to overcome a condition that has overwhelmed its defense mechanisms. Then the efforts of drugs or surgery may be warranted. When this occurs, your doctor of chiropractic will refer

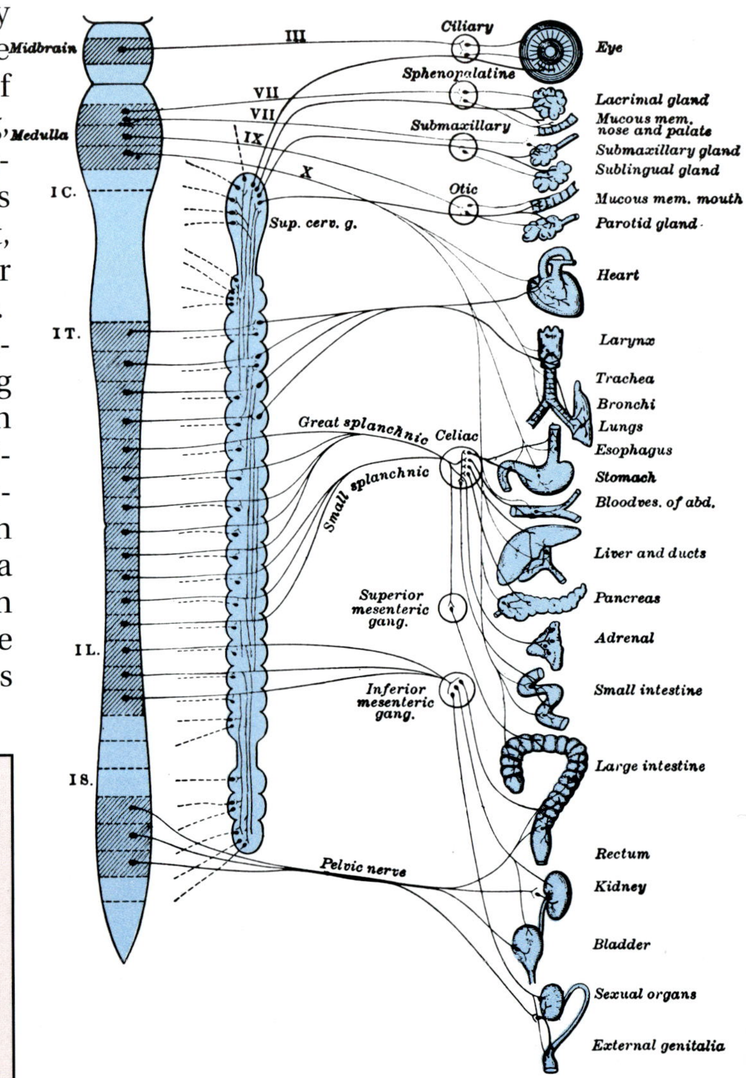

Figure 1

This illustration is taken from Gray's Anatomy[37], a standard textbook recognized and widely used in the leading schools of medicine, osteopathy and chiropractic. This is a schematic and does not accurately portray all of the details of the distribution of the efferent portions of the autonomic nervous system. More accurate information about the autonomic nervous system can be found in the chapter about the subject in Gray's Anatomy. Another excellent source for this information is in the chapter written by Cramer, G.D., Darby, S.A., Basic and Clinical Anatomy of the Spine, Spinal Cord and ANS, St. Louis: Mosby 1995.

you to the appropriate type of health practitioner for your particular problem. Your doctor's training enables him or her to advise you in these matters, so feel free to discuss your health problems at any time.

Many people think that chiropractors treat mainly orthopedic type conditions, such as backache, sciatica, shoulder/neck/arm pain, headache, whiplash and disc problems.[20,21,22,23,24,25,26,27,28,29,30,31,32] It is true that for these conditions one should try chiropractic first. The art of manipulation of the spine has been valued by patients and doctors since the time of Hippocrates. Other functional disorders such as those that involve organs and internal glands of the body may also, in some cases, respond to chiropractic care.[33,34,35,36] The significance of the nervous system in maintaining health suggests that conditions which are not responding to conventional care, may benefit from a short-term trial of chiropractic care. Your doctor of chiropractic would be pleased to discuss your conditions with you to determine if care may be appropriate in your individual case.

How Is Evaluation By A Doctor Of Chiropractic Unique?

First of all, your patient history will identify the chief complaint that encouraged you to visit your chiropractor. As a patient you might also be asked about your family history, dietary habits, other treatment you may have had (chiropractic, osteopathic, medical and other), your job, and other questions, designed to help determine the nature of your illness and the state of your health. In addition to the consultation, case history, and physical examination, laboratory testing and x-ray examination may be performed in accordance with your doctor's clinical judgment. In addition, a careful spinal examination and analysis will be performed to detect any structural abnormalities. You may not see any connection between a fall 25 years ago, an accident as a child, or some other seemingly unrelated event and your present illness, but all these factors will be significant to your doctor of chiropractic when your total health profile is evaluated.

In some cases, spinal x-rays may be necessary. While much can be determined from a case history and physical examination, the x-ray enables your doctor to view the specific outline of your spinal column.

Much has been written warning against the over-utilization of x-rays. However, this information should not discourage comprehensive diagnostic procedures when needed to deal with your health problems. The truth is that all x-ray procedures should be used with caution and good judgment. Many facilities today employ special filtration devices to significantly reduce radiation exposure.[38] Your doctor of chiropractic is acutely aware of the concerns regarding over-radiation, and will determine if the benefits of x-ray outweigh the potential harm of such an examination.

Additionally, your doctor of chiropractic will most likely seek to identify spinal

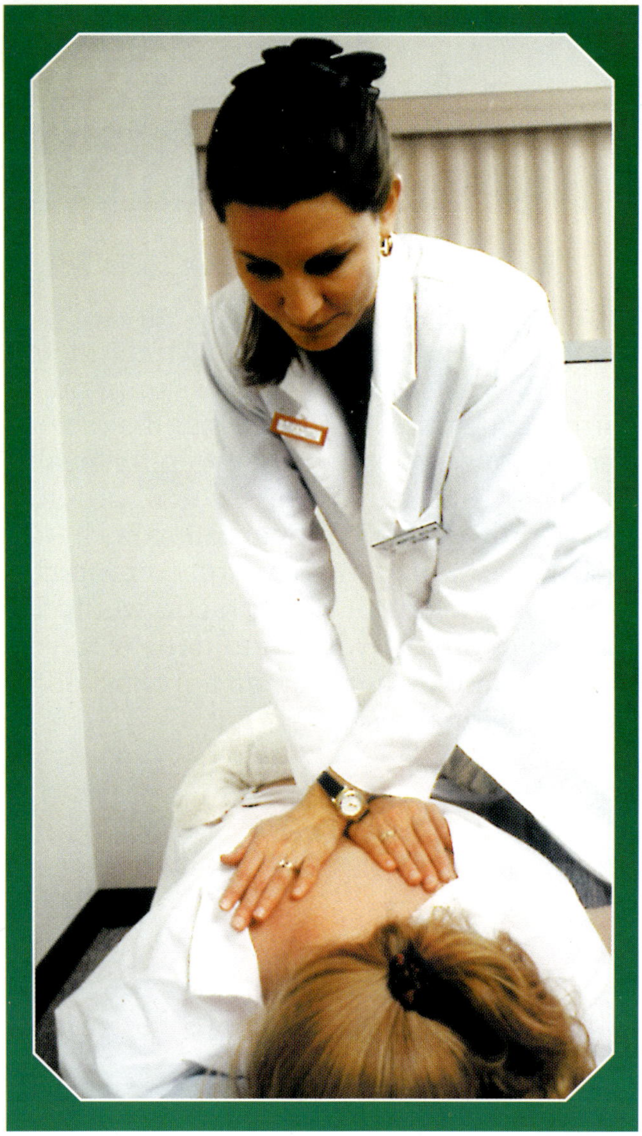

derangements through a gentle contact procedure known as motion palpation. This technique, coupled with a thorough understanding of spinal bio-mechanics, enables your doctor to identify areas of spinal stress and abnormal movement.[39,40,41,42]

Your spinal examination, and other physical examination findings, when analyzed through the skill and experience of your chiropractor, greatly aids in the identification of problem areas in the musculoskeletal system which may be contributing to your health ailment. The spinal analysis is one of the basic examinations used in evaluating your health problem from a structural point of view, and for determining if it is appropriate to begin chiropractic care.

How Does A Doctor Of Chiropractic Adjust My Spine?

"An adjustment," as doctors of chiropractic use the term, means the specific manipulation of one or more spinal or other malfunctioning joints (articulations). These abnormalities within the spinal column may cause irritability within the nervous system and interfere with normal nerve supply. Doctors of chiropractic spend years learning to examine the spine and understand the complex motions of the vertebrae. Additionally, they learn to administer a specific spinal adjustment. Considerable skill and dexterity are required to become proficient in the art of chiropractic adjusting.

If you remember the theory of chiropractic — that many ailments may come about as a result of improper nerve innervation — you will understand why your doctor will do everything he or she can to restore proper nerve function and proper structural mobility to your body.

The primary treatment by your doctor will be specific vertebral adjustments or "manipulations," as they are sometimes called. Particular attention will be paid to that area of your spine where a spinal subluxation (dysfunction or lesion) has been detected. Once these spinal areas have been adjusted (manipulated) to restore normal movement, the resulting change may have a positive influence on your area of complaint or discomfort.

The adjustment is usually given by hand. It consists of placing the patient on a precisely designed adjusting table, or chair, or other equipment, and then applying pressure, using specialized chiropractic techniques, to the areas of the spine that are out of proper alignment or that do not move properly within their normal range of motion.[43,44,45]

Doctors of chiropractic employ a wide variety of treatment methods, and the specific procedure to be used will be determined following a careful evaluation of your physical examination, case history and other findings.[46,47,48,49]

The experience of your doctor in manipulative procedures will determine the type of manipulation and the frequency with which you will be manipulated. The number of treatments required by each patient may vary to some degree, depending on the severity and duration of your problem.[50,51] Your doctor has available a variety of measurements and patient questionnaires designed to monitor your progress.[15,16]

How Long Will I Take To Improve?

There is no definite answer to that question since every case is different. Your doctor has treated numerous other patients with similar problems, and in many cases will be able to give you an estimate of the time it will take to expect results.

In most instances, the patient's concept of "being well" is to be free of symptoms that caused the patient to come to the doctor's office in the first place. It is common for a person to come to a doctor of chiropractic after having spent weeks in pain while seeking relief with drugs and other types of therapy. If that approach proves ineffective, the patient seeks chiropractic treatment, often as a last resort.

After receiving a careful examination and adjustments, if needed, to remove nerve irritation, some patients feel significant improvement rather quickly. It is often natural for such patients to think they are already well. There is, however, much more to illness than pain.

Patients should ask these questions: "Why did I get sick in the first place?" "What caused this problem to develop?" "Is it possible that this problem has been developing for a long time?" "How can I avoid these problems in the future?" Doctors of chiropractic teach that we should try to determine the underlying cause of the problem and attempt to correct it, rather than trying to remove the symptoms and have you "think" you are well.

How long it will take to actually "get well" or improve depends on many factors such as lifestyle, weight, age, and how long the condition has been present. Other factors such as living habits, occupation, genetics, attitude, and of course your cooperation, will all contribute to the time required for you to improve. Your doctor of chiropractic will suggest an individualized program designed to help your recovery in the shortest possible time, and then show you how to stay that way.

This booklet has been prepared to give you a basic understanding of chiropractic. Should you have additional questions, please do not hesitate to inquire. Through a frank discussion of your health problems, your doctor of chiropractic can help you learn about your health, and how to maintain it.

Will Supportive Therapy Be Used With My Condition?

The spinal adjustment (manipulation) is a predominant factor in providing chiropractic care for your condition. The adjustment, however, may not be the only procedure your chiropractor may employ in the course of your care and case management.[52,53]

The chiropractic profession utilized drugless therapeutics (natural therapies) as early as 1903.[54] Natural agents such as heat, cold, water, light, and exercise, are some of the drugless measures which are available to humans in abundant quantities. When controlled, these elements may exert a beneficial influence on body function. There are other forms of physiologic therapeutics which involve electrical stimulation, ultrasound, traction, postural support (cervical support pillows and flexible, custom-made foot orthotics), dietary management and other natural procedures which are known to have specific physiological influence on the body. These may or may not be utilized by your doctor in the course of your case management depending upon your needs. These natural agents are basically measures used to influence the body. Utilizing specific adjustments (manipulations) in conjunction with these procedures, your doctor of chiropractic's goal is to remove structural or nerve irritation which can be a major contributing factor in your health ailment.

Structural interferences may be caused by falls, strains, sprains, body blows, distortions, faulty posture, or trauma. Such interferences often cause postural misalignments. Regaining postural stability may require supportive therapy at the foundation of your body — your feet — with the application of flexible, custom-made spinal/pelvic stabilizers (foot orthotics). Negative attitudes, harmful living habits and other factors may also adversely affect the normal performance of muscles, organs, and other body functions.

In the course of your treatment, your doctor may recommend some procedures which you should employ at home, such as a cervical support pillow and/or rehabilitative therapeutic exercise with equipment designed for your specific conditional needs. If so, follow the instructions carefully and utilize only those procedures recommended, and only in the manner prescribed. By so doing, you will assure the fastest and most effective results.

Can Nutritional Supplements Help?

There can be no reasonable doubt that nutrition plays a vital role in the maintenance of a positive state of health and the prevention and treatment of disease. When proper diet and nutrients are supplied to the tissues of the body, they exert powerful influences on body metabolism.

Your doctor may suggest certain herbal products or specific nutritional products for you. These products are not without the potential for harmful side effects, especially if used improperly. All products you ingest, whether recommended or purchased by you independently should be discussed with your doctor. He or she may recommend a particular supplement product to help fulfill your individual need and complement your overall health care program. Patient's with special needs, such as women who require additional amounts of calcium and vitamin D (to prevent a negative calcium balance which results in a loss of bone strength) are a good example.[55]

To quote the Select Committee on Nutritional and Human Needs, "In the view of many doctors and nutritionists consulted by the Select Committee, changes in diet amount to a wave of malnutrition of both over-and under-consumption that may be as profoundly damaging as the widespread contagious diseases of the early part of the century."[56]

Vitamins, minerals, herbs, and similar products are considered essential by some leading authorities. Many consider vitamins and minerals, when taken properly, to be vital ingredients to maintain a healthy body. Nutritional supplements help the body increase resistance to fight infection, promote healing, improve joint motion, support nerve function and improve many other vital body processes. It is important that you obtain current information concerning herbs, vitamins and minerals and be aware of the value and risks associated with

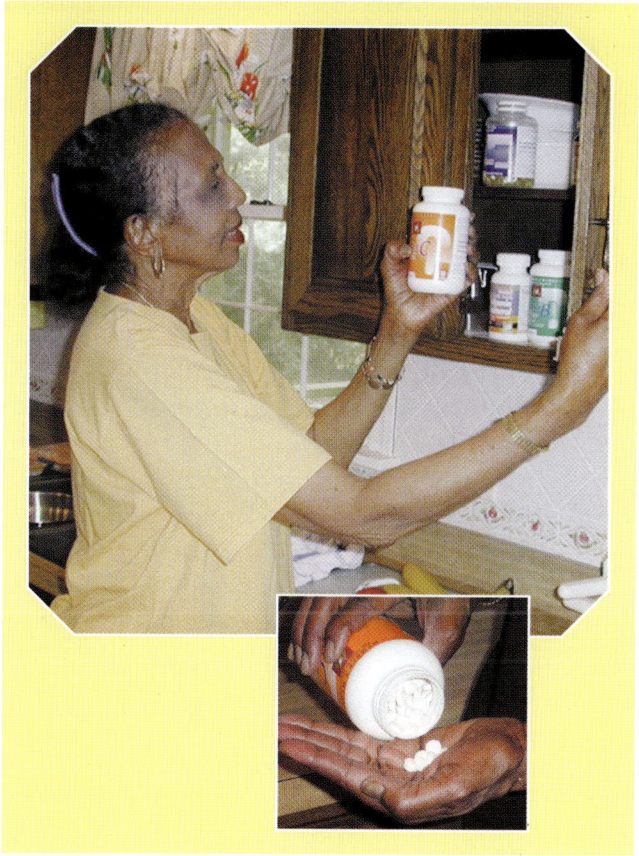

supplements when you add them to your diet.[57,58] Your doctor of chiropractic has had considerable training in nutrition and can help you avoid any toxic effects or adverse interaction of improper consumption of nutritional substances. If you have any questions about your nutritional needs, consult your chiropractor for more specific information and advice.

Proper nutrition and the intake of vitamins should be reviewed with your doctor. There are also many internet sites which can provide additional information. We offer several websites which may provide helpful information.

www.intelihealth.com/IH/ihtIH

www.nutrition.gov

Some Circumstances Which May Require Supplements

1. Use of oral contraceptives or estrogen-replacement compounds, pregnancy, and women breast-feeding.
2. Drug therapy which may interfere with the absorption of nutrients: i.e., antibiotics, diuretics, steroids.
3. Alcoholism.
4. Individuals who are dieting.
5. Cancer — including cancer therapies, e.g., radiation and chemotherapy.
6. Any major trauma or physical disease, e.g., severe burns.
7. Age specific poor diet profiles: i.e. Seniors and Teenagers whose dietary habits are often inadequate to maintain health.

This list was compiled from *Nutritional Support In Medical Practice,* Anderson et al, Harper & Rowe Publishers, Hagerstown, MD.

Your Diet And Your Health

The subject of diet deserves your most careful attention. Nutritional needs are often misunderstood by patients who wish to lose weight.

When your chiropractor says that you must have proper nutrition, you may be thinking of three ample meals daily; of meat, bread, potatoes, a dessert, and a drink. You need them, or some of them, but they are only a small part of real nutrition.

When your doctor speaks of nutrition, he or she is also referring to minerals and vitamins, and wholesome foods. He or she is talking about the raw materials which nature requires for continuously building and rebuilding the cells of your body.

Some of these properties are in all foods, though it is possible to destroy or diminish their value by improper cooking. Others are very scarce and can be obtained only from certain fresh vegetables, fruits, or from the parts of meat that few of us eat.

The so-called "balanced diet" does not exist, in reality, due to the variety of processes which food undergoes from the time of planting until it reaches your table.[57] To get as close as possible to a balanced diet, we suggest the following:

1. Eat plenty of fruits, vegetables, and whole grains, which are good sources of vitamins and minerals. When vegetables are stewed, save the stock for soups. The mineral values are more likely to be in the broth than in the food. Grains supply complex carbohydrates for energy and may be beneficial in the prevention of cardiovascular disease, intestinal disease and adult onset diabetes.[62]
2. Balance your intake of carefully selected lean beef, pork, lamb, veal, chicken, turkey, and fish, which are all part of the "MEAT" group. Limit your intake of fat and saturated fatty acids.[63] Studies show that people with high density lipoprotein (HDL) [the good guys] and low levels of LDL [the bad guys] are much less likely to develop heart disease.[64]
3. Eat less sugar and foods high in sugar content. Sugar has been implicated in health problems from tooth decay to obesity, from heart disease to diabetes.[65] Pastries and pies can be eaten in moderation by a healthy person; too much is never advisable. They should not be eaten by anyone who is in poor health or who has a weak digestive system. Fresh fruits, or simple custards are preferable.
4. Decrease salt consumption and foods high in salt content. Some authorities believe salt intake is one factor in some patients with high blood pressure.[66]

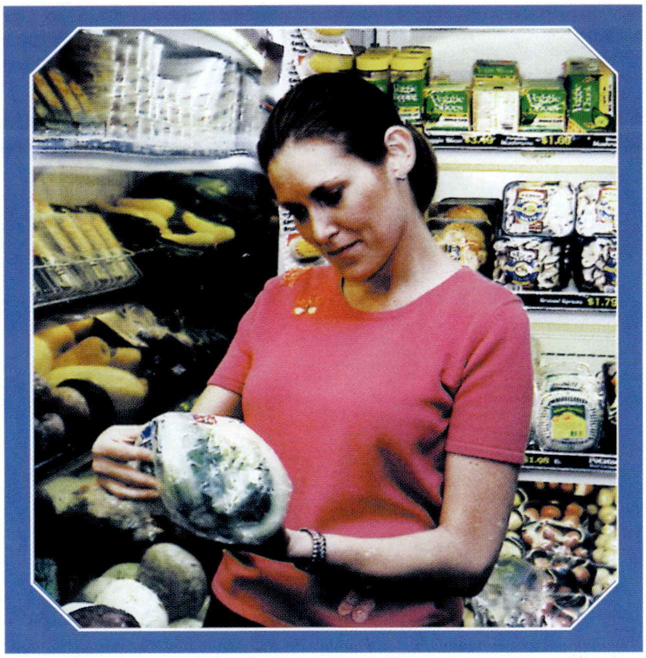

An excess of tea and coffee is discouraged. Water or fruit juices, with little or no sugar, are more healthful drinks for most people. Stay away from all tobacco products, as their direct and indirect influence on health is no longer in question.

We offer this quick list of food items which should be greatly reduced in our daily intake.

* White refined sugar and white refined flour
* Alcoholic beverages, coffee, and "cola" drinks
* Artificially flavored products with many added preservatives
* "Junk foods", candy and empty calorie snacks
* Foods high in saturated fat, and fried foods including many "fast foods"
* Convenience type foods are often low in nutritional value.

This list is not all-inclusive, but should serve as a guide for those individuals who are sincerely interested in their health and well-being. For those individuals wanting to find out more about nutrition and health matters, the American Dietetic Association has a website, www.eatright.org, which can be accessed for more information.

What About Those Miracle Diets?

Many people seeking to lose weight are lured by the promises of "quick fixes." Food fads, "wonder" diets promising a "new slim you," are promoted daily in hour-long infomercials. Promises about diets that sound too good to be true are rampant. Unhealthy eating habits begin early in life and often continue into adulthood. The working mother and dad coupled with a hectic schedule of activities for youngsters make it difficult for wholesome meals to become part of an everyday routine.

It is important, however, not to be lured by the promises of weight loss that involve drugs having many far-reaching harmful effects. Equally as important is the harm you can cause to your body by engaging in potentially harmful dieting activities. Fad diets and quick weight loss schemes could be harmful if not monitored. It is important that you discuss your weight reduction and exercise program with your chiropractor.

In most instances, the answer to quick diet schemes is an emphatic "NO." An improper diet is a significant factor in many human ailments.[68]

We have become so conditioned by advertising that we begin to think that junk foods are the norm, and those who advocate healthy diets, raw vegetables, vitamins, and proper balanced nutrition, are the nutritional "nuts." It is recommended that you maintain a sensible approach to your diet.

This booklet is not intended to replace the sound advice of your doctor, but merely intended to make you aware of sound nutritional information essential to your good health.

The Following Publications And Organizations May Provide Helpful Information:

1. *Prevention,* Rodale Press, Inc., 33 East Minor Street, Emmaus, PA 18049, www.rodalepress.com
2. *Food and Nutrition Information Center,* National Agricultural Library, Room 105, 10301 Baltimore Avenue, Beltsville, MD 20705-2351, www.nal.usda.gov/fnic/
3. *Weight Watchers, International,* 175 Crossways Park West, Woodbury, NY 11797 www.weightwatchers.com
4. *Permanent Weight Loss Cassette,* Program by Dr. Clark Cameron, available from Nightingale-Conant, 7300 N. Lehigh, Niles, IL 60714 www.nightingale-conant.com
5. *Recipes for Fat Controlled Low Cholesterol Meals,* American Heart Association, 7272 Greenville Avenue, Dallas, TX 75231.
6. *A Guide for Weight Reduction.* American Heart Association www.americanheart.org
7. There are many websites which can be used to obtain good information relative to your health. Several we suggest are as follows: www.news@EDIETS.com
8. www.healthfinder.gov

The Weight Problem

Remember, the spine is held in place by ligaments and muscles which must be maintained in a state of balance and proper tone. Obesity can cause an imbalance in your body structures.

The doctor of chiropractic pays special attention to your weight and posture because of the importance they play in helping to maintain a properly balanced spinal column. Being overweight can delay your ability to respond to the care you are receiving. If your doctor considers this to be a major factor in your condition he or she may provide you with a diet or other suggestions on how to lose weight. These may include psychological counseling, behavior modification, hypnosis, or a supervised weight reduction program.

Weight imbalance not only increases spinal problems but adds greatly to the increase of heart disease, hypertension (high blood pressure), circulatory disorders, and many other ills which are steadily increasing. Overweight is not confined to adults and "heavy children usually become heavy adults."[67]

Our emphasis must shift from the *"quantity"* to the *"quality"* of food we consume. With proper knowledge of food and food products, the entire health of our population will be improved. Some conditions of obesity are hormonal and should be appropriated treated. In such cases, specific laboratory studies may be necessary to properly evaluate the condition. Your doctor will determine if these are warranted. In most instances, however, overweight is the result of too much food intake. Other important factors such as improper eating habits, inadequate exercise, and sedentary work and leisure activities, all play critical roles in an individual remaining overweight. Developing a positive mental attitude and a firm commitment to changing bad life style habits are needed to overcome the problem of overweight.

Should you have a specific question concerning your weight, ask your doctor for information and advice before you begin any program.

Water Intake

The body is wonderfully complex and unique and needs water among other things in order to function properly. Most of us do not drink enough water. Generally speaking, adults should drink at least six to eight glasses of liquid daily: most of us can stand more. Certain kinds of bladder and kidney difficulties may alter this amount.

The vital need for water is not fully appreciated by most people. Most of the major systems of the body need water to function properly. Your skin, which covers the entire body, loses water every day through perspiration. The lungs require approximately two glasses of water each day to function properly. The small intestines also need water for optimum function to promote proper elimination.

Kidneys, which are very important organs in the body's elimination system, utilize a large quantity of water daily to carry out wastes.

Many people use thirst as the primary criterion for regulating their water intake; this is not a valid indicator. The body needs fluid whether you have a desire for it or not. To provide a consistent supply throughout the day, regular consumption is best. A routine for example could incorporate a glass of cool, but not iced, water when you get up in the morning. This should precede breakfast by some 10-15 minutes. Water, coupled with moderate exercise, will greatly aid in activating the intestinal tract and help to establish normal elimination.

Many people today drink bottled water or have filtration or purification devices to help filter out impurities. This is an excellent idea. Additionally, water should be tested at least annually for impurities or contaminants, particularly if derived from a source that is not regularly monitored, such as a well.

Regularity

The body must dispose of the wastes that it cannot use. These wastes putrefy and decompose if retained in the body too long, which may be detrimental to health. Therefore, elimination should be regular.

Elimination is accomplished through four systems: the skin, lungs, kidneys and the bowels. If the suggestions in this booklet as to exercise, fresh air, and water are followed, there will usually be little difficulty with the elimination through the first three systems. Bowel elimination requires special attention.

Daily bowel elimination is important. A person should try to establish a habit of maintaining a predictable schedule for this purpose, such as just before retiring or right after breakfast. Water, exercise and a wise choice of foods are important for regular bowel elimination.

Maintaining a regularity of bowel elimination may be aided by eating natural "bran" or high fiber foods such as potatoes, peas, beans, fresh fruits and vegetables. This high fiber diet has proven extremely effective for many people by providing the intestinal tract with "bulk" or roughage. A daily routine of adding several tablespoons of natural bran to your cereal will greatly aid in maintaining and promoting better elimination. Recent studies have shown that this is very beneficial to those who have conditions such as diverticular disease.[59]

Posture And Your Health

The spine is not an inflexible rod as some people would believe. In fact, it is quite flexible. Structurally strong, it allows the agile movement of the human body. It not only supports the body and all its organs, it also protects the sensitive and delicate spinal cord and spinal nerves. Every activity, even breathing, demands movement of the spine, ribs and attachments. The spine gives the human structure both strength and agility.[69]

Humans are one of a small group of beings who are classified as "biped" (stand erect on two legs). While this particular position gives humans the advantages of agility, leverage and mobility, it also creates certain structural stresses. The continual pull of gravity can cause postural imbalances in the feet. Because the human body is like a chain of interconnected links (weightbearing joints), improper movements at the lowest link (the foot/ankle) can cause abnormal movement or twisting at other such links higher up — the knee, hip, pelvis, and spine. These abnormal joint motions often produce stress pain. So even if your feet don't hurt, they may be contributing to pain in another part of your body. Flexible, custom-made orthotics are designed to work with chiropractic adjustments to help restore postural balance and relieve pain.

The most obvious benefit of good posture is efficiency and comfort. Yet, because of the interrelationship of the structural (bone) and functional (organ) systems of the body, posture is also a factor which can impact health. For example, poor posture compromises the movements of the rib cage and does not allow the lungs to function at maximum efficiency in order to bring much needed oxygen to the tissue and eliminate carbon dioxide wastes. Other vital organs of the body are also restricted when body posture is improper, producing structural stress.[70]

Your doctor of chiropractic is a specialist in body mechanics, and places considerable emphasis on the body's structural, muscular, and neurological components. Additionally, the holistic (wellness) approach of chiropractic care includes training in nutrition, disease prevention, life-style intervention, and the psychological aspects that play a vital role in health. Because there is considerable emphasis on the structural, muscular and neurological aspects and how they relate to health, the focus is aimed at maintaining sound body mechanics and good posture.

The Importance Of Posture To Physical Development

While people with good posture stand straighter and look better, there are advantages to correct posture that go beyond appearance.

The human body, like a machine, to function properly is dependent on balance, rhythm, timing and coordinated action of all its components. Correct posture enables the body to function more efficiently.

Can Posture Affect Mental Attitude?

Posture affects how others see you and as you see yourself. It reflects your personality, your confidence, your attitude, your ability...and your health.

There is an interrelationship between how you stand, sit and walk, and how you feel. More than anything else, it is a tip-off to others as to whether you are a positive person or a negative person, a strong person or a weak person, a healthy person or an ill person.

Many Postural Faults Can Be Helped

The effects of poor posture can be serious in terms of health, comfort and efficiency, causing fatigue. Many problems can be helped. If you or a member of your family have what appears to be a postural problem, you should seek the advice of a doctor of chiropractic. Unless there is an anatomical (structural deformity) or pathological (dis-

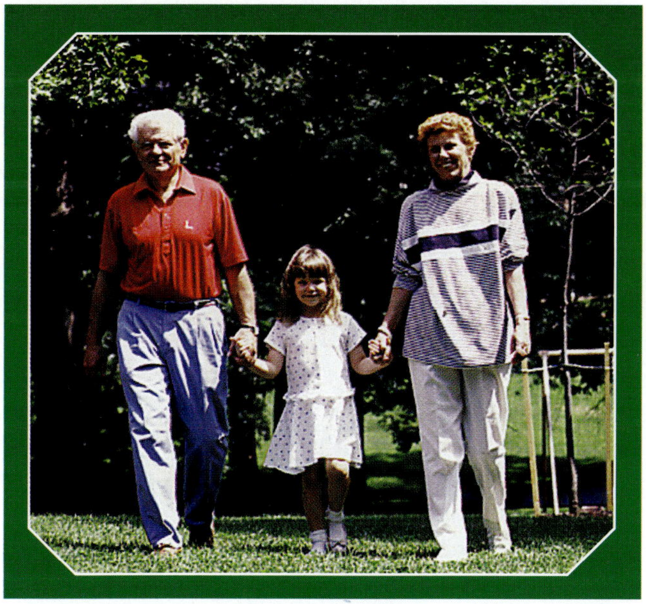

ease-caused) disturbance, the chances for correction are excellent.[43,71]

If not corrected, poor posture can affect the health and well-being of the individual throughout his or her life. Poor posture contributes to shallow breathing, a cramped chest cavity, faulty digestion, poor elimination; and poor circulation, each of which affects not only the functions of individual organs, but also the system. It will also contribute to the accelerated degeneration of spinal and other joints and discs. Lack of energy and reduced coordination are just two of many symptoms of a body that is not functioning efficiently.

Check Your Posture

Poor posture may be caused by scoliosis which is a lateral or side-bending of the spine. This condition often becomes pronounced and creates a mechanical disadvantage to the spine and supporting structures. Many cases of scoliosis are detected through junior and high school spinal screening examinations. Your doctor of chiropractic should be consulted if there is any indication that a scoliosis may be present. Many cases of scoliosis can be helped with conservative measures such as spinal adjustments and rehabilitative exercises.[43] If further evaluation is warranted, your doctor of chiropractic will refer you to the appropriate facility.

What Causes Poor Posture?

There are many reasons for poor posture, the most serious of which is a birth defect. In most cases, a combination of factors causes poor posture. Some of the more obvious are:

1. Visual problems.
2. Emotional problems.
3. Excessive weight.
4. Foot problems or improper shoes.
5. Weak muscles, muscle imbalance.
6. Improper nutrition.
7. Poor sleep support (mattress).
8. Injury to muscles, ligaments, tendons or bones.
9. Negative mental and physical attitudes.
10. Occupational stress.

What Are Some Benefits Of Correct Posture?

1. Improves your health.
2. Improves your appearance.
3. Improves your coordination.
4. Increases your strength.
5. Gives you more stamina.
6. Makes your clothing fit better.
7. Gives you confidence.
8. Gives you better body balance and makes you more agile.
9. Reduces the possibility of injury.
10. Aids in physical and mental development.

Your Feet Affect Your Posture And Your Health

If your feet are somehow contributing to your postural problem, your chiropractor may need to perform corrective adjustments as well as suggest custom orthotics to help absorb shock, maintain balance and eliminate fatigue. For more information on orthotics:
www.footlevelers.com

Chiropractic Care For Children

New patients, in a chiropractor's office, who see an infant or young child, often comment: "I didn't know you treated children!" It really shouldn't be so surprising, the spine is subject to stress and strain from the very moment of birth. Birth itself is probably the first shock to the spine and nervous system that the infant receives. Think about the pressure on the infant at the time of delivery and the potential pull on the infant's head and neck even during a normal, uncomplicated delivery.

We have always been told to use caution when holding a baby. That's because the child's neck is very weak. The muscles have not developed sufficiently to hold the head erect. The very weight of the child's head is more than the neck muscles can carry.

As the child develops, there is the usual progression of crawling, walking, running and other activities. During childhood activities, how often have we witnessed a child fall? In fact, there are many falls which occur while simply learning to walk. Because of the elasticity of youth, a child is able to bounce back again. But there is always the question, "Was there any harm done?"

The chiropractic profession places considerable emphasis on structural balance and has attributed considerable importance to the potential problems which can result from these seemingly harmless childhood incidents. The profession has maintained that these seemingly minor accidents are an element to consider in the health of our youngsters.

We have limited this booklet only to the mechanical and structural imbalances which relate to your child's health. There are, obviously, other factors that can influence and impact upon a child's health. We have attempted to illustrate the importance of maintaining a properly functioning nervous system that allows the body to perform at its maximum capacity. The strains to which children are subjected, can easily be a contributing factor in creating spinal subluxations (malfunctions) and /or nerve irritation. Throughout this introduction booklet, we have tried to demonstrate that many conditions can be caused by spinal derangements producing irritations to the nervous system. Common disorders of childhood such as colds, constipation, asthma, colic, enuresis (bedwetting), and ear infections (otitis media), may be helped through spinal adjustments (manipulations) and conservative chiropractic management.[23,24,72,73]

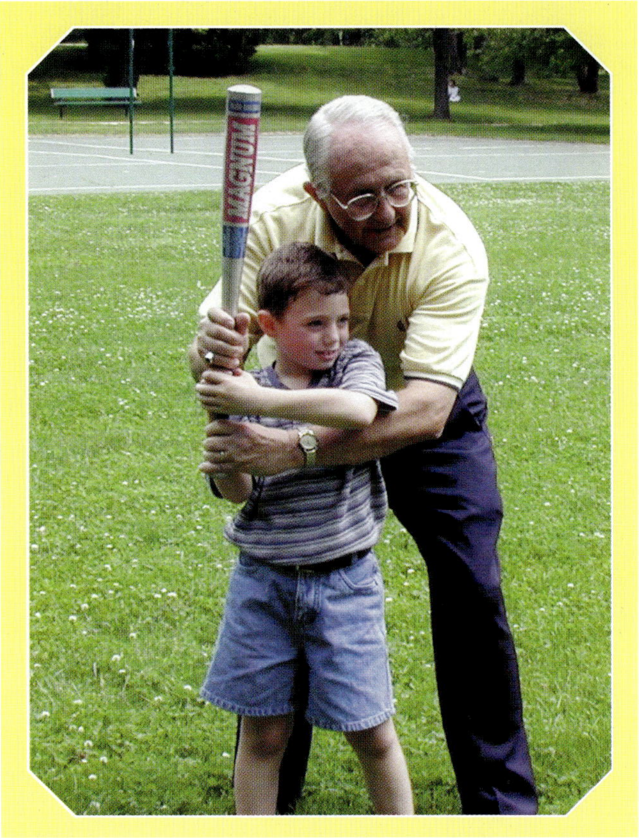

Not all conditions will respond to conservative chiropractic management and your doctor of chiropractic is fully trained to recognize when referral and/or other interventions are needed.

Some childhood conditions, such as functional scoliosis (spinal curvature), which may be correctable with chiropractic care, are too often neglected and plague the child throughout his or her lifetime. Many of your neighbors and friends have their children's spines checked by a doctor of chiropractic because it gives them confidence and reassurance. The consideration of chiropractic care for your child is reasonable and logical. If parents were as concerned about having their children's spines checked for minor derangements (subluxations) as they are about having their children's teeth checked for cavities, they would be helping their youngsters to attain a healthier state of well-being. Proper spinal care is important to your child's health. Don't neglect a spinal examination in his or her next health check-up.

Chiropractic Care For Senior Citizens

The prime objective of chiropractic care discussed throughout this booklet is to optimize human health by keeping the nervous system free from interference, thus allowing the body to function at its maximum capacity.

The advisability of chiropractic care for many conditions has been suggested. It has been pointed out that while some conditions may not seem to be directly related to the spine, theories have suggested that some conditions may be linked to a spinal or neurological factor and may explain why these conditions respond to chiropractic adjustments.

Why the need for chiropractic care for our senior citizens? Aging is a natural and normal process which each person must undergo. Older patients are subjected to structural problems such as degenerative joint disease (arthritis) and, therefore, many of their ailments are related to the spine and extremities. Pain and stiffness are two of the most frequent complaints of the senior citizen.[74]

Why this happens is easily understood: the elastic discs and supporting ligaments have lost much of their ability to stretch and move due to aging, and are therefore less flexible.

As a person ages, the muscles which help to maintain the spine in its normal alignment begin to lose the tone needed to maintain balance. When this occurs, the spinal vertebrae have a greater tendency to slip or move erratically. This affects the spinal nerves which lead to vital parts of the body.

Another condition often affecting senior citizens is osteoporosis. This occurs mainly in women after menopause, and is characterized by thinning of bones leaving them fragile and susceptible to fractures. Almost one out of every four women over 65 develops an osteoporotic fracture. Factors contributing to osteoporosis are hormone loss, lack of physical activity, calcium deficiency, alcohol, cigarette smoking, and certain medications. Talk to your doctor about making some decisions on how to effectively cope with osteoporosis. Your lifestyle is important and you can do many things to help you live with osteoporosis and to help prevent injury.

Earlier in this booklet, it was pointed out that chiropractic adjustments (manipulations) of spinal joint derangements may help the body to retain and maintain its normal balance and mobility.

Chronic conditions associated with the process of aging, such as degenerative arthritis, circulatory disorders, constipation, and stiffness of various joints, may benefit from corrective spinal adjustments.[35]

The chiropractic profession has always focused a high degree of attention on the senior citizen. This has been done mainly because the senior citizen's happiness largely depends on physical health and mental attitude. The chiropractic profession has directed much of its attention towards making the older person better able to function as a vital member of society. In the past few years, several studies have been conducted which have focused on the health promotion and preventive attitudes of doctors of chiropractic. These studies have attempted to determine if maintenance care and health promotion services for chiropractic patients 65 years or older have been effective.[75] The studies suggest that there may be positive health benefits achieved by individuals who have received chiropractic care on a regular basis. There is also a growing positive trend toward health maintenance, evidenced by a reduction in smoking and a more cautious attitude about the use of prescription and over-the-counter drugs. Also an increase in exercise and healthy lifestyles, as well as a growing awareness concerning the value of nutritional requirements for health will enhance the quality of life for most senior citizens. Much of the new attitude is fueled by an increase in longevity and the general awareness of the direct effects lifestyle has on health.[75,76]

Chronic pain is a significant problem for many senior citizens. However, non-pharmacological (non-drug) approaches, oftentimes used alone or in combination with appropriate drug-based strategies, should be an integral part of health care plans for most chronic pain patients. Non-drug pain management strategies encompass a broad range of treatments and supportive physical modalities. Educational programs, acupuncture, acupressure, transcutaneous nerve stimulation (TENS), heat, cold, massage, relaxation, biofeedback, meditation, specific exercise, shiatsu massage, spiritual healing, and group therapy, have each in some instances been helpful for some patients. Moreover, these healthcare interventions carry minimal risk of adverse effects.[61]

Consult your doctor of chiropractic for a consultation and evaluation. Perhaps you can gain many more years of productive living through chiropractic health care. In many instances your quality of life may be significantly improved by including these reasonable approaches as part of your overall health program. Remember, "youth is a feeling and an attitude… not an age."

Facts About Discs

1. What Are Spinal Discs?

The discs within the spine are basically cartilage pads which separate, cushion, and help to bind together the twenty-four (24) vertebrae. These discs are part of a system much like the "suspension system" of your vehicle, in that they provide a cushioning effect and flexibility for your spine. It is these discs which allow you to move and bend your neck and back. It is important to remember that discs do not have a direct blood supply. They receive their nutrition by a pumping process called osmosis and diffusion resulting from the movement of vertebrae above and below the disc. When this "suspension" system is not working properly because of improper spinal motion, the nutrients are not supplied to the disc, and degeneration may result.

Lumbar Spine

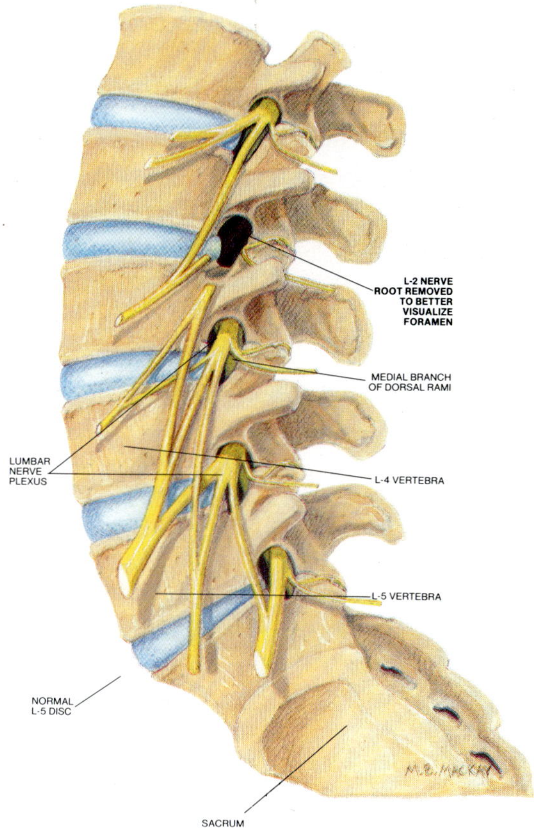

NORMAL LATERAL
(Low Back Side View)

Without the discs, the spine would be an inflexible solid mass of bone. Spinal discs make up approximately one-fourth of the length of the spine. Throughout your entire life, these discs are constantly exposed to compression, torque, twisting and injury, resulting in stress to the disc mechanism.

2. How Does an Injury ToThe Discs Occur?

Disc injury occurs as a result of many factors such as genetics and the normal "wear and tear" process of aging. Subluxations (minor displacements or functional disturbances) of the spine which were discussed earlier in this booklet are also a factor in the cause of disc injury.[77] The most common manner in which these displacements of the spine occur are through sudden, forceful movements of the spine, such as falling, lifting, twisting, auto accidents, or perhaps an unexpected slap on the neck or back. Sometimes, the mere position that the spine is in while performing a minor task can cause a disc injury. This can occur even when lifting a very light object.[74]

3. Facts About Herniated Discs.

Disc disease is the topic of considerable discussion today and terms such as ruptured, herniated, bulged, degenerated, and protruded are often used interchangeably; however, they are not the same. The spinal discs are constantly subject to gravity and torque from body movements and, therefore, are susceptible to degeneration from wear and tear. The terms "degenerative disc" or "degenerative joint disease" more accurately describe the "wear and tear" process which occurs. Derangements of the spine are a major contributing factor in back pain. Derangements (subluxations) or structural imbalances allow the disc to bulge, protrude, herniate, or impinge upon nerves. Sciatic pain is a common example of the possible irritation which can result from a degenerative or herniated disc.[77,78,79]

4. Back Surgery, Will It Be Necessary?

Many leading authorities state that only a small percentage of disc herniations actually require surgery. However, of those individuals, who are carefully and properly selected to be treated by surgical methods, the percentage of satisfactory results is good. By all indications, too many individuals are misdiagnosed as having a "herniated disc." These cases are too often improperly and aggressively managed. Many of these cases have resulted in considerable unnecessary and costly surgery, often with no positive outcome or resulting in a failed back syndrome. There are indications for surgery, which should be thoroughly understood and carefully considered. Intractable pain (pain which is not able to be relieved), recurrent crippling attacks of pain and immobility, which affect the livelihood of the individual and his or her "quality of life," and any

DISC PROTRUSION

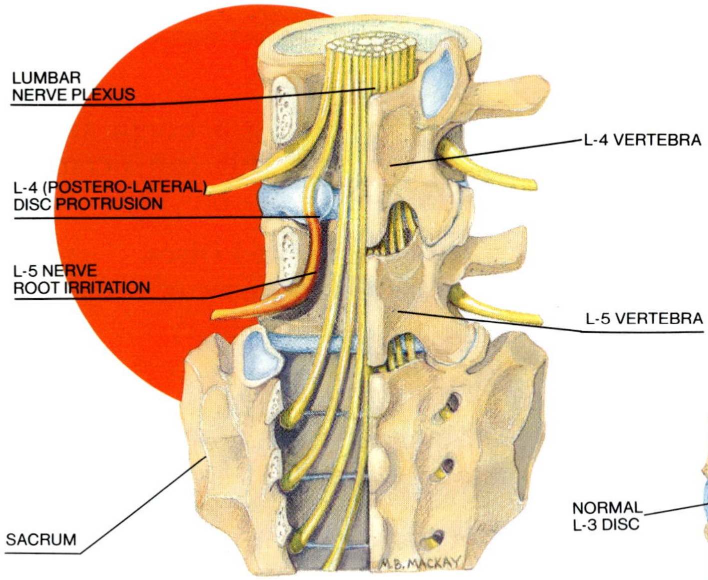

(P-A VIEW OF LUMBAR SPINE)

View of lumbo sacral spine with left portion of the posterior elements removed to visualize the postero-lateral L-4 disc protrusion and resulting irritation of the L-5 nerve root.

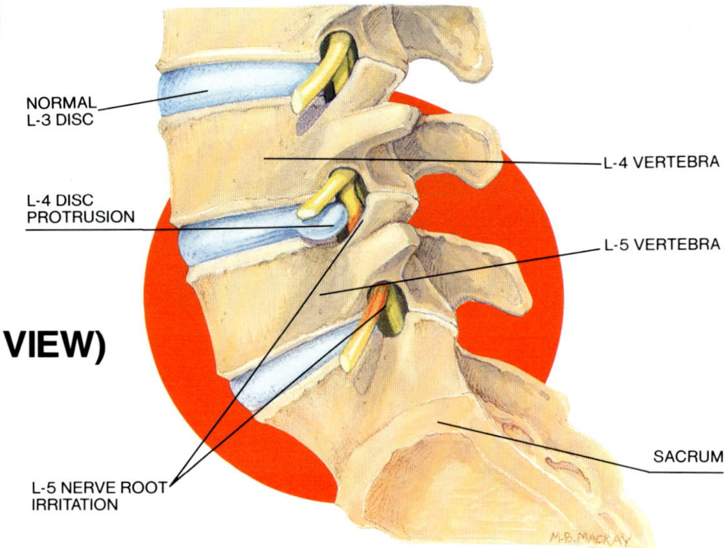

(SIDE VIEW)

SYMPTOMS AND SIGNS OF DISC PROTRUSION

- Deep, dull ache in low back.
- Deep, dull ache in buttocks and/or posterior thigh, calf and sometimes foot.
- Splinting muscle spasm of low back (reflex spasm immobilizing lumbar spine in antalgic position).
- Sharp pain in low back upon movement.
- Pain, loss of sensation, numbness and/or tingling in leg and/or foot.
- Muscle weakness.
- Inability to stand on toes or heels.
- Pain accentuated by forward bending, sneezing or straining.
- Bladder and bowel incontinence.
- Other symptoms may be present.
- Limited flexion and/or extrusion of back.
- Increased pain with prolonged sitting, standing or lying on stomach.
- Pain relieved when lying on back or side with knees and hips flexed.
- Difficult to rise from sitting or lying position.
- Coughing, sneezing or straining increases low back and/or leg pain.
- Pain and stiffness in morning (usually difficult to put on stockings and shoes).
- Increased pain after walking short distances (relieved with rest).
- Decrease or loss of knee or ankle reflexes.
- Muscle atrophy.
- Other signs may be present.

significant neurological deficit (loss) in ability to walk, properly balance, or the ability to control bowel or bladder functions, are signs of the need for a possible surgical consultation.[34] After careful evaluation of your problem, your doctor of chiropractic may advise you to consider a short-term trial of conservative chiropractic care. In the event this does not produce satisfactory results, you and your doctor will decide on a recommendation for a second opionion consultation prior to determining the need for surgery. While it is difficult to generalize about disc herniations, you should inform your doctor of any changes in your condition.

5. What To Do For Disc Problems

Clinical evidence suggests that many "disc herniations" can be successfully treated, and the resulting pain and muscle spasms effectively alleviated through the application of conservative chiropractic care. This may include specific spinal adjustments and, if appropriate, the use of supportive therapy.[80,81] A fact which is often overlooked is that muscle spasm and pain are your body's way of protecting you from further tissue damage. Often the conservative approach is not to attack the pain and spasm, but rather to determine and correct the reason for your pain and spasm. When this is accomplished, your pain and spasm will most likely diminish and eventually disappear. The doctor of chiropractic directs his or her efforts toward the skillful restoration of the vertebrae to their normal range of motion, thereby reducing inflammation, stress and pressure on the spinal discs and spinal joints.

The chiropractic profession is the leader in the field of manipulation and conservative management of disc injuries. The application of the principles of chiropractic spinal management can lessen the possibility of costly hospitalization, unnecessary surgery and its often negative after effects, and considerable pain.

There are thousands of unnecessary spinal surgeries performed each year in the United States, with sources estimating as many as 44,000.[92] A recent government report from the Agency for Health Care Policy and Research (AHCPR), which developed Guidelines For Acute Low Back Pain in Adults, suggested that the treating clinician discuss all treatment options with the patient. Surgery should be considered if the condition is disabling, the symptoms persist without improvement, or there is progressive deterioration in the condition. The study suggests that at least a one-month trial of conservative care be considered as a first treatment option.[82]

Among the recommended "preferred treatments" for acute low-back pain, spinal manipulation is one of the conservative methods indicated. Doctors of chiropractic perform 94% of all spinal manipulation administered in the United States.[93]

6. How Long Will A Disc Problem Take To Respond?

The length of time you have the condition can greatly affect your response time. If, for example, you have only been treated with physical therapy, muscle relaxants or pain medication, and your condition was the result of a spinal derangement, you will have allowed the condition to possibly become chronic, while you attempted to treat only the pain. Removal of the pain is not necessarily always beneficial; it is the body's "warning signal" to alert you to problems.

The chiropractic conservative approach to the management of disc herniations utilizes, if indicated, a careful and strict regimen of ice or heat when necessary, supportive therapy, special rehabilitative exercises and specific chiropractic adjustments (manipulations). Careful ongoing monitoring of your progress by your doctor of chiropractic, as well as your providing him or her with important information on your improvement, will be essential to the successful management of your condition.

Specific chiropractic adjustments may improve spinal mobility and unlock the facet joints (gliding joints of the spine which allow movement) helping to relieve the accompanying muscle, ligament and tendon contractions, as well as the mechanical or reflex irritation of the nerve roots. Some disc cases respond in one or two weeks. For some patients, however, it may take longer. In any case, it requires time to heal, even after the pain has been relieved.

Disc problems are "potential time bombs," which can go off at any time. You must use caution when lifting, bending or performing any task where extra physical exertion is required. The erect posture of the human spine, coupled with repeated minor trauma or injury, increases the susceptibility of the spine and discs to degeneration.

Low Back Pain— A Universal Problem

Osteoarthritis is commonly considered a "wear-and-tear" process and is associated with degenerative changes in the disc, which results in an altered relationship (derangement) between adjacent vertebrae.[83] This derangement causes an increased strain, as well as a loss of motion of the gliding joints of the spine. These gliding joints (facets) are found in pairs, along the entire spine, and their function is to allow for movement and flexibility of the spine. When these facet joints are affected by repeated trauma from excessive strenuous athletic activities, heredity, weakened or deconditioned muscles, and the inevitable aging process, low back and/or leg pain is commonly experienced.

Degenerative changes in the disc or an altered function in the facet joints, contribute significantly to the "wear-and-tear" process, placing a strain upon this important area of the spine.[84] The osteoarthritic spine becomes less flexible, and therefore becomes more vulnerable to injury. A simple

Lumbar Spine

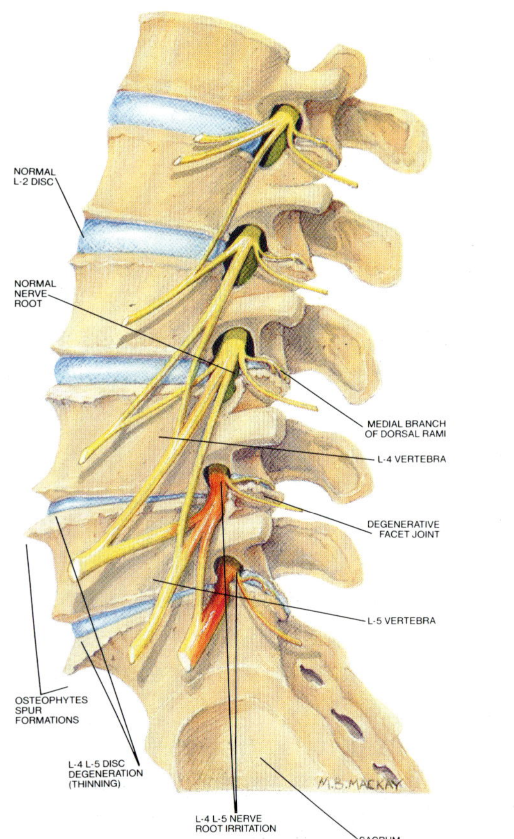

OSTEOARTHRITIS
DEGENERATIVE HYPERTROPHIC SPONDYLITIS
(Side View)

unexpected or forced movement, physically heavy work, improper posture, frequent bending or lifting all can produce strain and injury to these facet joints.[74,80,85]

Chiropractic care, which may include spinal adjustments (manipulations) and physiologic therapeutics such as ice, heat, ultrasound, galvanic and other electric stimulation, may help to reduce pain, and muscle spasm. It is important to follow the specific instructions of your doctor regarding your work activity, leisure activity, exercise program, weight control, occupational factors, and frequency of visits in order to achieve the optimum relief from your back pain and to help prevent recurrence.

SIGNS AND SYMPTOMS OF AN OSTEOARTHRITIC SPINE

- Limited movement in low back.
- Increased pain and stiffness in the morning or after sitting which improves with movement or activity.
- Tightness and cramping in buttocks and leg muscles.
- Recurrent, frequent bouts of low back and leg pain.
- Increased leg pain after walking short distances (relieved with rest).
- Other signs may be present.
- Dull, painfully stiff low backache.
- Frequent muscle spasms in low back.
- Numbness, tingling, and a feeling of weakness into legs and/or toes.
- Radiating pain into buttocks, legs and feet.
- Constant painful inability to walk or move without the use of some form of support.
- Other symptoms may be present.

Instructions For Home Care For A Low Back Injury

When convalescing from a back sprain or strain or acute disc injury, the following are recommended:

1. Do not apply heat unless instructed by your chiropractor.
2. Do not take hot tub baths with acute low back problems until instructed to do so.
3. Do not sleep on a soft bed. In most instances a firm bed is preferable. A tip when getting out of bed is to turn to your side, attempt to place your feet on the floor, push yourself to a sitting position, attempting to keep your back straight. This often helps to ease the distress of getting out of bed.
4. Do not sleep on your abdomen. Sleep on your side with one or both knees slightly bent. If you sleep on your back, place a pillow under your knees to relieve the strain on your lower back.
5. Do not sit on soft or deep chairs or sofas.
6. Do not walk up or down stairs more than absolutely necessary. Do not walk on rough terrain.
7. Do not lift heavy objects. When lifting, bring objects close to you, using your legs in lifting, not your back. Do not turn your head while lifting.
8. Do not stoop forward with knees straight. Squat down, using your knees and strong leg muscles, not your back.
9. Do not stand in one spot for long periods of time. If it is necessary, such as when ironing, keep one foot on a low stool to help relieve the strain to your low back. Alternate your right and left leg periodically. The stool can be 4" to 6" high and adjusted to your comfort.
10. Do not drive during the acute pain

state. Try to have a family member or friend drive you to the office until you ask your doctor about driving yourself.

11. Do not engage in any exercise program without consulting your doctor. *Back exercises are illustrated on pages 43-50.

12. If you are taking any over-the-counter medication or prescription pain medication, be certain to inform your doctor of chiropractic.

Should symptoms reoccur, or worsen, consult your chiropractor promptly.

What to Do For Sudden Back Injury

Many severe attacks of back pain develop from something as insignificant as bending over a bathroom sink, reaching to pick up some small item, sneezing, or reaching into low cabinets. Usually, a series of small incidents leads up to cause the back injury. Heavy lifting, falls or severe strain are early precipitating factors in many back injuries. Most patients will usually remember some incident after they have had time to think about past accidents, falls, or they have been reminded by family or friends.

Faulty spinal dynamics are often a cause of severe back pain. Faulty spinal alignment, over a period of time, will cause gradual weakening of disc fibers and other ligaments. In this weakened condition, sometimes all it may take to cause severe back pain is the leverage of a simple movement, such as reaching into the cupboard.

When such an incident occurs;

1. Lie down immediately in any position that is comfortable. Lying on your side with knees drawn up (fetal position) with a pillow between your knees provides a comfortable position. Care should be taken to keep your neck in line with the rest of your spine.
2. Use ice. If you do not have a soft gel ice pack, you can use an item from your freezer. Even more helpful is to freeze water in a styrofoam cup and peel away an inch of the cup and rub the ice over the injured area as an ice massage. Use the ice for 20-30 minutes. This may hurt at first, but after several minutes, the area will become desensitized and you will feel less discomfort. Utilizing ice for less than 15 minutes will significantly diminish the effectiveness. Reapply ice as directed. Do not keep ice directly on the area for longer than 30 minutes as this will impair circulation and cause additional complications.
3. Call your doctor of chiropractic and make arrangements to go to the office as soon as possible. In some cases, it may be suggested that you remain at home and use some "first aid" measures suggested by your doctor, such as ice applications, massage, supports, simple exercises or other suggestions based upon your doctor's recommendations.
4. Do not sit in a soft recliner or soft sofa or overstuffed chair, as this may aggravate your condition and make it difficult for you to get out of the chair. It is advisable to use a straight back chair with two arms to provide support getting into and out of the chair. A small pillow behind your low back may provide some additional comfort.
5. A walker is very helpful in providing support and balance while standing and walking.
6. Maintain a positive outlook. Conservative chiropractic care is very effective in many back injury conditions. However, it takes time for the body to heal, so be patient.

We suggest you visit the website www.spine-health.com for additional information on back and neck pain.

Care Of The Cervical Spine (Neck)

Minor neck aches, pain and stiffness are something we all suffer with from time to time. Such annoyances are usually brought on by overwork or holding the head in an awkward position, such as sleeping upright in a chair. Fortunately, these are minor situations and clear up after a day of rest or a good night's sleep.

On the other hand, recurring aches, pains and stiffness of the neck, or discomfort that lasts more than twenty-four hours, should have professional evaluation. Persistent pain in the neck is a symptom of something gone wrong. Repeated episodes of stiff neck may indicate early stages of joint or disc degeneration.[86,87]

The neck (cervical spine) contains the upper portion of the spinal cord and eight pairs of spinal nerves. The nerves of the cervical spine which are "pinched," or have pressure on them, can produce symptoms in various parts of the body. For example, pain between the shoulder blades and some arm complaints originate in the neck.

In addition to pain and stiffness, symptoms that may be caused by problems in the cervical (neck) spine can include: headache; dizziness; pain in the face, ears and scalp; pain in the shoulder-arm-hand; numbness and tingling in one or more of the fingers; throat discomfort; difficulty in breathing; and chest pains, to name some of the more common complaints.[87,88] The neck is the most vulnerable part of the spinal column, subject to all sorts of major and minor injuries. It is composed of seven small bones (vertebrae) and supported by only muscles and ligaments which must hold and balance

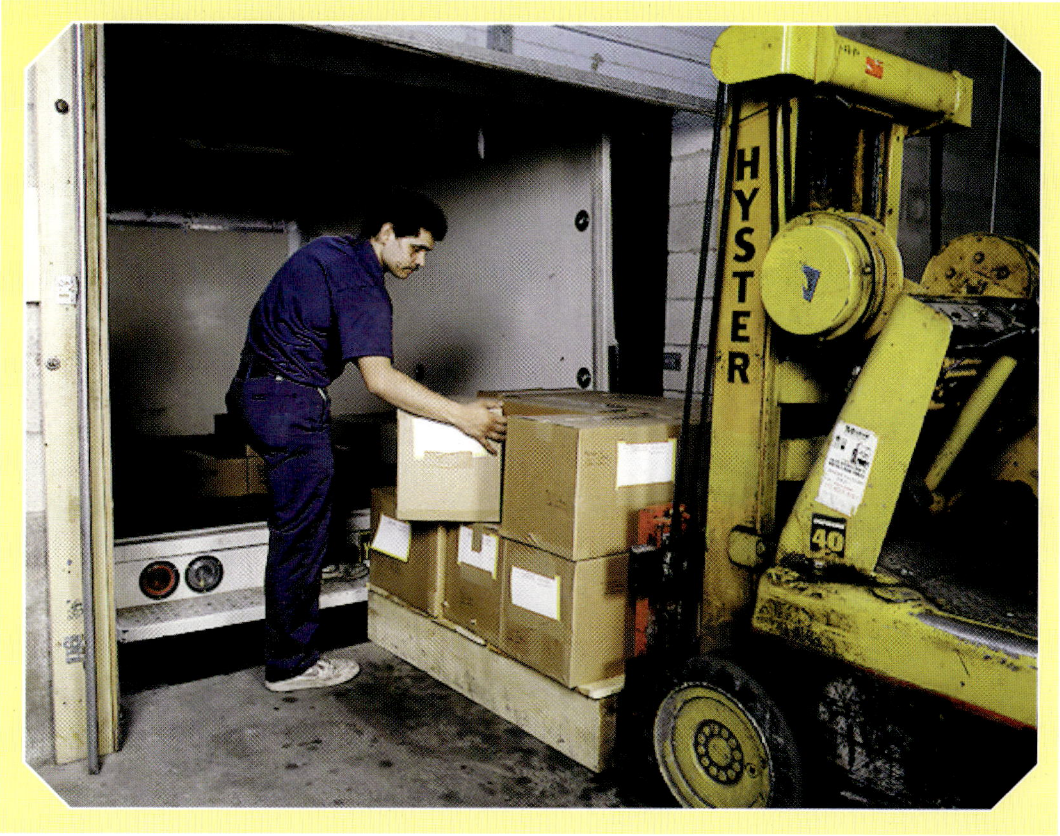

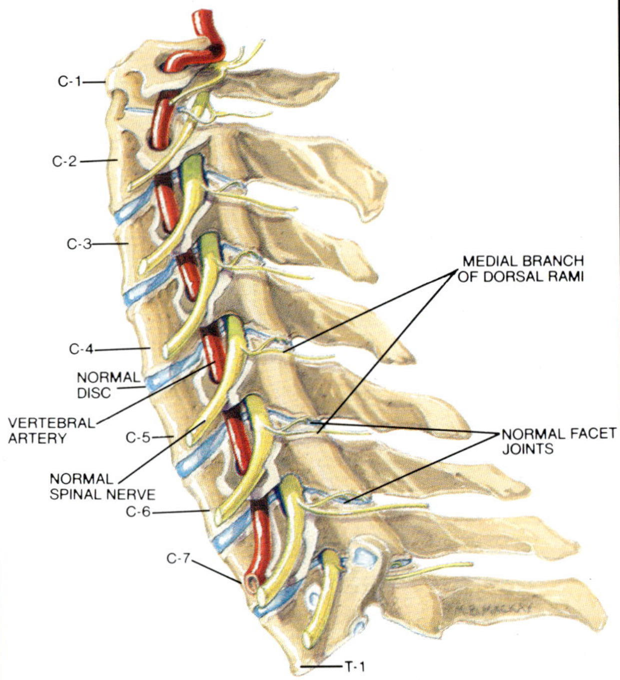

NORMAL CERVICAL SPINE

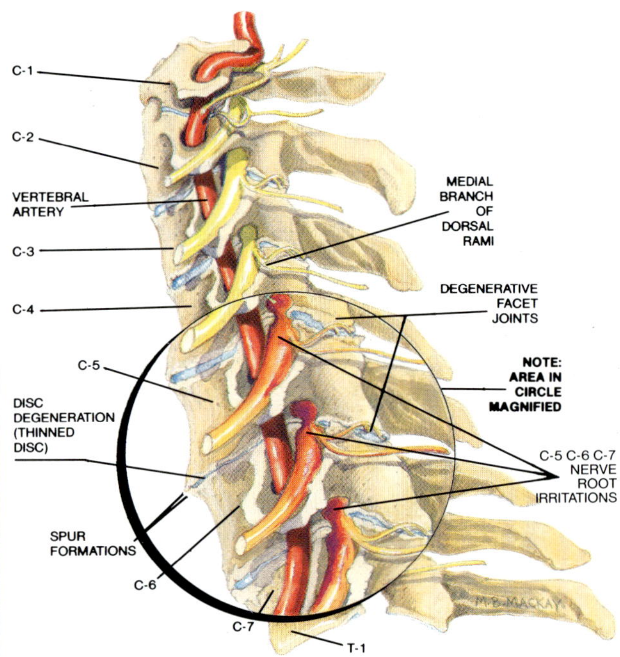

OSTEOARTHRITIS
SEVERE DEGENERATIVE CHANGES

a head which weighs approximately ten pounds.

The neck is very susceptible to stresses and strains from any source and will often react violently to seemingly insignificant falls or accidents. According to some authorities, the neck is strained more frequently than any other structure in the body.

Common Causes of Neck Strain:

1. Bad posture — forward thrusted head with chin pointed up.
2. Overwork — continuing to work beyond endurance.
3. Muscular weakness.
4. Nervous and emotional tension.
5. Underlying disease, such as arthritis.
6. Accidents — falls or automobile "whiplash" injuries.
7. Military-type posture.

The type of discomfort or pattern of pain sometimes serves as a clue to what is wrong.

For example:

1. A neck that is relatively pain-free in the morning and worsens as the day goes on, frequently indicates strain, fatigue or muscular weakness.
2. A neck that is stiff and painful in the morning and feels better as the day goes on, may indicate some underlying condition such as arthritis.
3. Neck pain that is aggravated by coughing or sneezing may indicate a disc herniation.
4. Dizziness, light-headedness, or pain that develops when the head is turned or elevated, is evidence of a possible vascular problem. However, symptoms of lightheadedness, vertigo, unsteadiness, weakness, difficulty with balance also can be caused by an imbalance in the cervical (neck) spine. These symptoms when properly evaluated will determine the need for additional testing, referral, or the appropriateness of chiropractic conservative intervention.

Allow your doctor of chiropractic to determine what your needs are. His or her training will determine if you need additional specialized examination procedures such as, MRI, CT scan, EMG, Ultrasound or other specific testing to confirm the exact nature of your neck problem.

Too often, a patient considers repeated episodes of a stiff neck as something very minor and expects one office visit to correct the entire problem. Sometimes this may be true, but more often and realistically the cause of the discomfort may require additional care and follow-up.

Management of the overall problem of a neck disorder should be supervised by your chiropractor. The care of structural defects, a disease process, cervical instability, etc., requires professional evaluation and supervision. This cannot be over-emphasized!

In addition to treatment for the specific condition, your doctor of chiropractic may recommend exercises to restore normal range of motion or to overcome muscular weakness, which can cause neck pain. Proper exercise may greatly help to alleviate aches, pains, tensions, and nerve irritations that may have developed as a result of strain, disease, injuries, or lack of use.

Weak muscles must struggle to get a person through the day, while well-toned muscles allow one to work and play without tiring. Exercising will develop more efficient muscles by improving tone and strengthening the muscles connected to the cervical spine. Ask your doctor of chiropractic about specific muscle strengthening exercises.

Range of motion exercises, while not designed to strengthen muscles, are an excellent means of helping to restore the normal motion to the joints of the cervical spine. This is especially important if an arthritic type condition is present. The key to joint function is mobility, flexibility and strength.

Once your neck problem has been brought under control, it is up to you to follow your doctor's advice on how to avoid further strain and acquire a stronger neck.

Note: See Exercise section to follow starting on page 43.

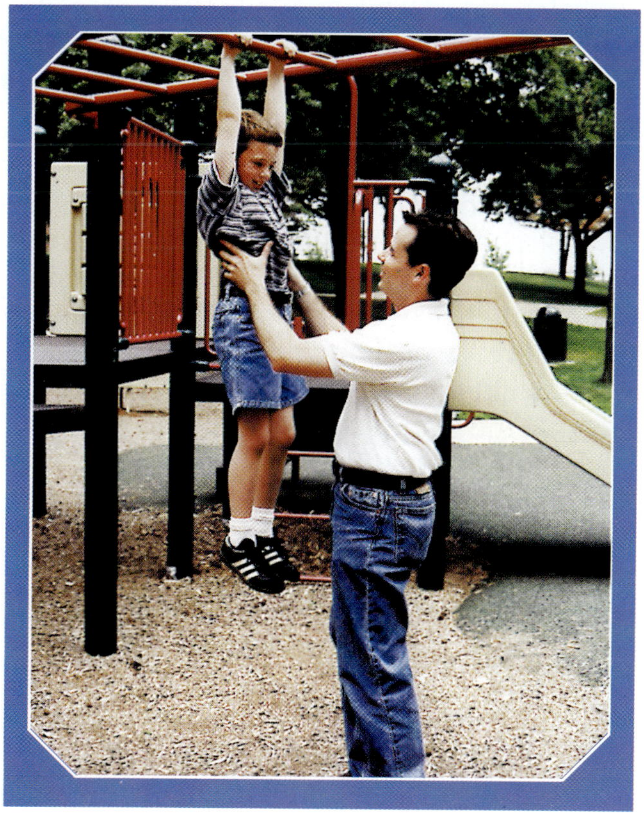

"Whiplash" Injury

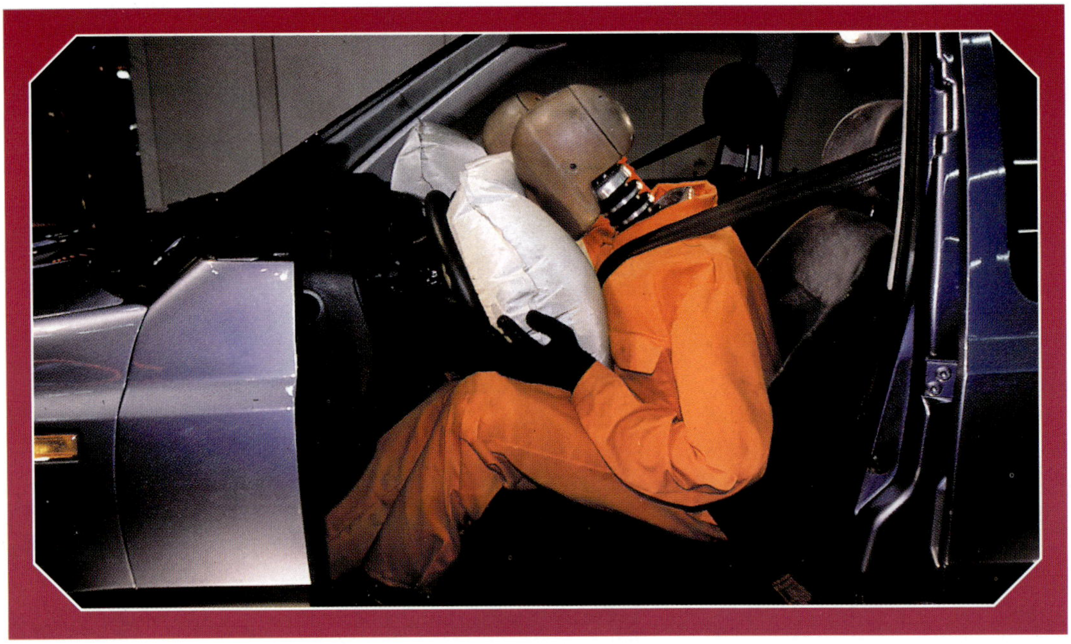

Whiplash Associated Disorders (WAD), or "Whiplash," is the common name given to an injury where there is a hyperextension (increased backward motion), hyperflexion (increased forward motion) injury to the cervical (neck) spine. Its name comes from the fact that the spine is held in place in the mid-back by the attachment of the rib cage. Any movement, therefore, to which the spine may be subjected, as in the case of an auto accident, or severe fall, commonly results in the neck being "whipped" forward or backward or sideways in relationship to the rib cage.

The cervical spine described earlier in this booklet outlines some of the potential ailments which can occur to the neck. A typical example of a common injury to the neck region is illustrated in the rear-end auto collision. The driver, not suspecting such an incident, is relaxed. The force from behind causes the head to quickly flip backwards and then thrust forward by the deceleration (quick stopping) motion.

This type of rapid movement and the manner in which the head is thrust about has been termed "whiplash." Many injuries of this nature are not immediately felt by the injured person. Authorities estimate that the injuries may not be felt for several hours, days and in rare cases even months or years following the incident.[88,89]

Examples of reactions from an injury of this nature could be: headaches, visual disturbance, stiffness of the neck, restriction of movement, shoulder, neck and arm pain, and neuralgia, to name but a few.[88,89]

Many victims attempt to treat the neck injury with home remedies increasing the possibility of further injury.

It is absolutely essential to have an examination by a doctor who is trained to examine the spine and related structures, and who understands the dynamics of the "whiplash" injury in order to rule out, or diminish, future problems.

The immediate damage to the muscles and ligaments will heal with scar formation if not treated properly. The healing will result in tissues that do not have the same elastic property or ability to stretch and therefore pain associated with the injury may continue.[90] The tearing of the ligaments and the trauma to the cervical spine (neck vertebrae) can result in significant spinal derangements, which left undetected and uncorrected, will result in degenerative changes to the neck region, and more specifically the discs.[86]

Chiropractic doctors are particularly concerned with the structural balance of the spine and nervous system. Careful attention is paid to proper alignment and mobility of the spine. Should you become involved in any accident or fall in which you suspect that your spine, particularly your neck, may have received a strain/ sprain injury, consult your doctor of chiropractic for an examination.

Prompt attention to any neck injury may help to avoid many of the symptoms which could develop at a later date and not be as readily treatable.

SIGNS AND SYMPTOMS EXPERIENCED BY PERSONS INJURED IN "WHIPLASH" TYPE INCIDENTS

- Stiffness/general achiness.
- Shoulder/neck/arm pain.
- Vertigo/dizziness.
- Numbness/tingling/weakness.
- Visual disturbances.
- Nausea/vomiting.
- Chest pain.
- Blood pressure irregularities
- Emotional complaints.
- The list is not exhaustive and all symptoms should be reported to your doctor.

INJURY TO THE CERVICAL SPINE

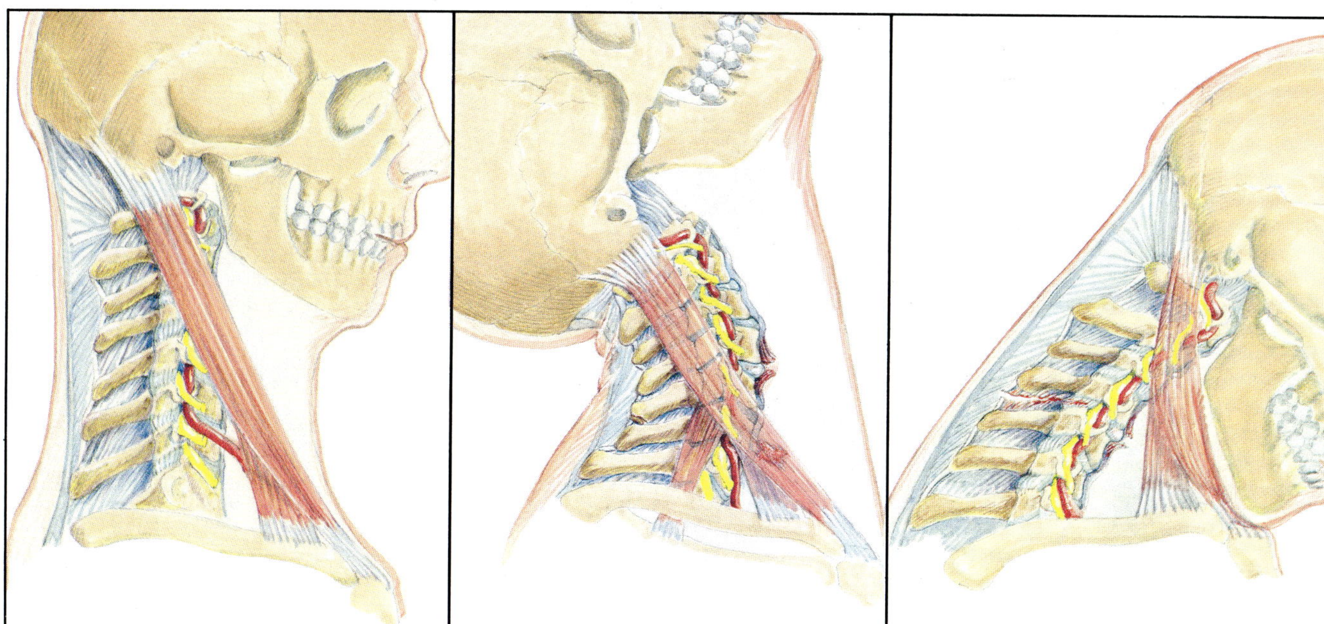

AT IMPACT

Lower body moves forward suddenly, head remains momentarily in place. Note loss of cervical curve.

HYPEREXTENSION

Head arcs backward upon the neck, protective flexor muscles contract.

HYPERFLEXION

Head rebounds forward, neck structures compress.

HYPEREXTENSION (REAR-END COLLISION)

VARIOUS INJURIES WHICH CAN RESULT FROM A "WHIPLASH" TYPE TRAUMA TO THE SPINE

- Vertebral dysfunction (Subluxation).
- Strain/sprain to the flexor and extensor muscle groups.
- Tearing of the retaining ligaments including portions of the discs of the spine.
- Herniation of the intervertebral disc.
- Intracranial trauma and concussion.
- Injury to other spinal areas.
- Vertebral artery trauma.
- Various fractures of the vertebra.
- Spinal cord and nerve injury.
- There may be other injuries which will necessitate further evaluation by your doctor.

OSTEOARTHRITIS COMMON SYMPTOMS OF DEGENERATIVE CHANGE IN THE CERVICAL SPINE (NECK)

- Neck pain.
- Headaches.
- Grating sensation when turning head and neck.
- Shoulder cap/neck/arm pain.
- Numbness and tingling into arm/hand/fingers.
- Lack of muscle coordination.
- Weak grip strength.
- Dizziness.
- Other symptoms may be present and should be discussed with your doctor.

Instructions For Home Care For A Neck Injury

1. Do not apply heat or massage with liniment unless instructed to do so by your doctor.
2. If support is needed, fold a towel until you can wrap it around your neck to form a support type collar. Do not use when lying down.
3. Avoid turning and bending neck in any type of motion that causes pain.
4. Avoid prolonged periods of sitting or standing in one position. Lie on back with small pillow under cervical spine (neck) for support.
5. If blurred vision, dizziness, headaches, ringing in ears, or nausea are experienced, contact your doctor immediately. If any of the above symptoms persist, avoid putting the head and neck in a position which will require extension of the neck (looking up) and rotation (looking over shoulder). If symptoms worsen and you are unable to contact a doctor, consult your nearest hospital emergency room for advice.
6. Instructions which apply to sudden back injury can also be used for sudden neck injury as it applies to ice application. (No. 2-3, page 32)

Is There A Reaction Following An Adjustment

In the course of being treated for spinal derangements (subluxations), there are certain reactions which you may experience. The most common is a slight aching or soreness in the spinal joints or muscles. This is due, in part, to the spinal joints beginning to once again move within their normal range of motion. Do not become alarmed if you experience this type of reaction. Our experience suggests this is a natural tissue response to an adjustment.

Reactions following a chiropractic adjustment vary greatly from person to person. These may vary from a great sense of exhilaration and well-being to the reaction described above. Most reactions usually will subside within several days and if they do not, you should report these to your doctor.

If you have any questions or any unusual reactions which concern you, do not hesitate to ask your doctor on your next visit or call the office for additional information.

Keeping Your Appointments

You should maintain your schedule of visits with your doctor of chiropractic. This is essential so he or she can give proper attention to your case. Best results can be obtained with mutual cooperation. If you are sincere in your desire to achieve improvement in your condition, following a carefully designed program will enhance your potential for achieving excellent results.

Your doctor will do his or her utmost to accommodate you with your appointments. A notice of twenty-four hours, if possible, should be given in the event you are unable to keep your scheduled visit.

It is essential that you keep your appointments, especially in the initial stage of your care. Health requires time and careful attention. Your cooperation is the best way to ensure the maximum benefit from your regimen of care.

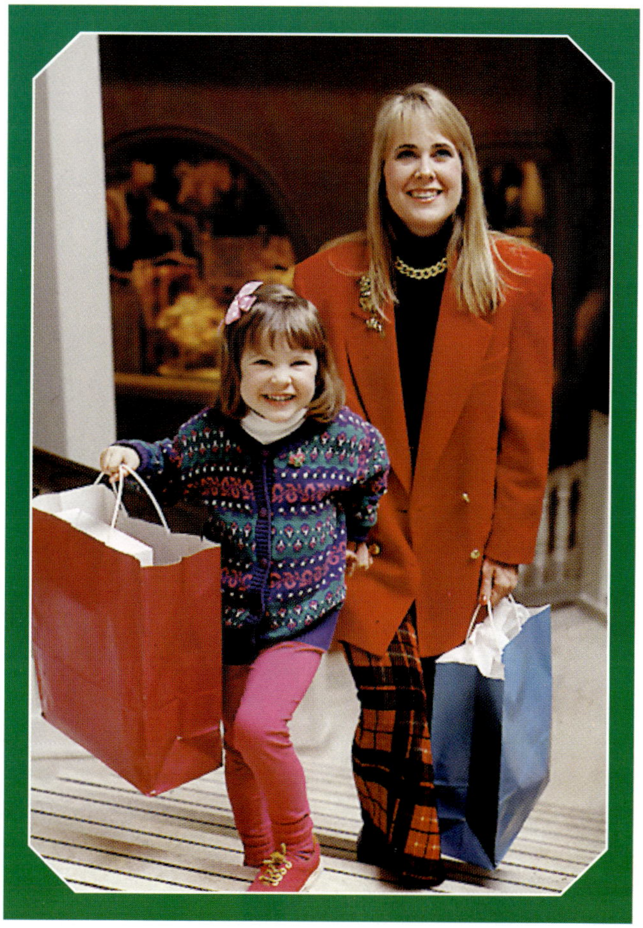

Personal Advice From Friends And Relatives

Direct personal referral from satisfied patients is still the number one way most people initially seek care from a doctor of chiropractic. However, there are many well-meaning friends and relatives who have not personally experienced the benefits of chiropractic care and may attempt to discourage you from consulting a doctor of chiropractic. It is difficult enough to be sick, without being subjected to doubts placed in your mind by well-meaning friends or relatives. Often these doubts are due to a lack of information or understanding regarding the chiropractic approach to health care. Since you have placed your confidence in your doctor, please allow him or her to advise you on matters relating to your treatment.

Chiropractic is not a panacea for all the ailments of humankind, and should not be viewed as such. In many instances, however, chiropractic represents a significant form of health care worthy of serious consideration by those individuals with conditions that may respond favorably and more effectively with chiropractic management. In many instances, particularly as they relate to the spine and musculoskeletal system, chiropractic is used as the primary form of care. In other instances, chiropractic may be used in conjunction with or complementary to other health care interventions.

Please read this booklet carefully and if you have any questions, ask your doctor.

The health care delivery system is becoming more complex and more demanding. It is the intent of this booklet to help explain and illustrate the science, philosophy and art of chiropractic. Chiropractic places considerable emphasis on "prevention." It is your chiropractor's goal to offer you sound advice and effective treatment so that you can enjoy better health.

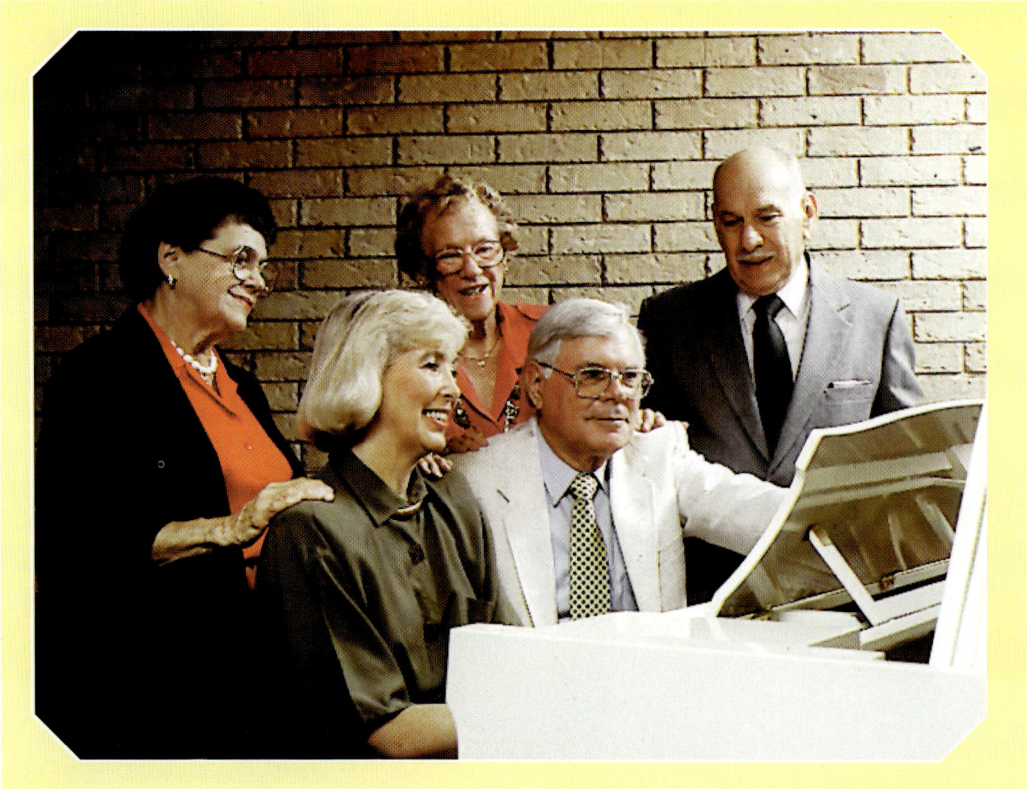

Exercise

Before beginning any exercise program, please consult with your doctor to be certain that you receive specific instructions on proper exercise for your state of health. Get a reasonable amount of exercise daily. This does not mean that you should immediately rush out to play a vigorous game of racquetball or tennis, or decide to run a marathon. Walking is an excellent form of exercise and can be done by almost everybody. There are other activities which provide some exercise such as "walking up those stairs" rather than using the elevator, "pushing" yourself away from the table before you eat that second helping. So are many forms of work or light household tasks.

Exercise is necessary for proper digestion and elimination. Exercise will keep your muscles toned, and promote better circulation, especially to the heart. You will find, in the next section of this booklet, some very carefully designed exercises for your back and neck. Your doctor will outline a special program for you.

Because exercise is essential to good health and to overcome certain muscular weaknesses, your doctor may prescribe specific exercises. These are a vital and important part of your therapy; do not forget them. Some exercises are designed to strengthen the muscles of your spine, so that spinal derangements (subluxations) may be minimized. If you neglect the exercises prescribed for you, you neglect an important part of your health regimen.

Health authorities are now questioning the wisdom and value of certain exercises.[52,60] Therefore, it is wise to be certain that you are indeed performing the proper exercises for your particular needs. The last section of this booklet is designed to aid you in exercising during your acute, sub-acute, and recovery stages. Do not do any exercise without consulting with your doctor first, and do only those exercises suggested. As your condition warrants, your doctor will suggest additional exercises to aid your rehabilitation.

Lack of proper exercise causes the muscles of your body to become weak and deconditioned. A muscle not used for a short period of time will begin to lose tone and strength. Exercise will prevent this wasting or atrophy of muscle, as well as releasing the body's endorphins (those feel-good chemicals) that will put you in a positive and pleasurable state of mind.

Research has shown that moderate exercise at least three times a week can increase your life span by at least two and one half years. Aerobic exercise is important and a program tailored to your weight, age and physical condition should be designed.[61,91] Scheduling a regular time for your workout can have surprising effects. People who exercise in the morning seem to be the most consistent. Exercising before the evening meal has the greatest benefit if weight loss is desired. The most important consideration is working the program into your schedule so that it becomes an important and pleasurable part of your daily routine. No matter when or how you exercise, be certain to discuss the kind of exercise and how you should approach exercising with your doctor. Exercise and physical fitness are extremely important.

For additional information on becoming fit, we recommend website www.shapeup.org.

Exercises For A Healthier Back And Neck

Treat Exercise With Respect

The following pages present helpful exercises for your neck and back.

While exercise has therapeutic benefits, it can have a reverse effect if not done with care and good judgment. It is best to follow a program outlined by your doctor of chiropractic which allows him or her to professionally monitor your progress.

Following are some important points to remember:

1. Wear clothes that will not impede or restrict your movements in any direction. Sweatsuits, leotards or loose clothing are best.
2. It is essential that you "warm-up" before engaging in an exercise session. Allow the muscles to loosen up before embarking on strenuous exercise by beginning each exercise session with a stretching routine. Applying heat or hot tub soak for five to ten minutes just before starting can help relax tight muscles.
3. Start by doing the movements slowly and carefully. As you gain confidence and strength, you may increase the speed along with the frequency, but speed is not essential! It is important to maintain a balanced breathing cycle with each exercise, inhaling and exhaling in rhythm.
4. Don't over-exercise, especially at the beginning. Do *only* the amount recommended by your doctor of chiropractic. Do only the exercises your doctor has recommended and in the order advised.
5. Floor exercises should be done on a firm, padded surface, such as a carpeted floor. If it is difficult getting down and up from the floor initially, a firm bed might be preferred. A small pillow under the head is sometimes more comfortable.

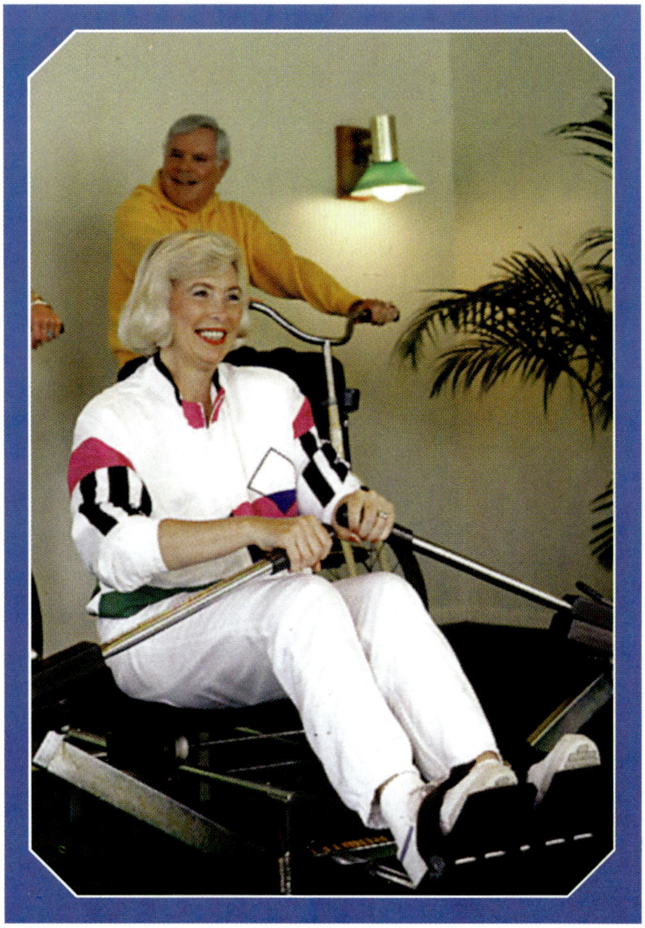

6. Exercise according to the routine recommended by your doctor of chiropractic. Do not skip a day and then try to make it up with heavier exercise. Sporadic exercising can be harmful.
7. If you feel slight discomfort during your exercises, do not become alarmed. This should disappear as your muscles become stronger and more conditioned to the routine. However, pain or discomfort should not persist. If it does, stop the routine and consult your doctor of chiropractic.
8. IMPORTANT: Follow directions precisely. It is important to avoid doing any type of exercise other than those recommended, particularly if you're recovering from a back or neck ailment.

Exercising To Rehabilitate And Strengthen The Low Back

Most low back pain patients experience three general stages before maximum recovery and rehabilitation is reached:

Stage 1—Acute/Pain Stage
Stage 2—Subacute/Recovery Stage
Stage 3—Chronic/Rehabilitative

Stage 1—Acute Pain Stage
(Signs and Symptoms)

- Low back pain
- Hip pain
- Leg pain
- Splinting muscle spasm
- Antalgic (bent) posture
- Muscle weakness
- Inability to stand on heels or toes
- Aggravated by sitting, standing, bending, coughing, sneezing, straining
- Difficulty in rising from a sitting or lying position

Stage 2—Subacute Recovery Stage

This stage is when the majority of signs and symptoms from the acute stage have subsided. You may continue to experience a dull, aching sensation in your low back, hips or legs, and possibly have a weak feeling in the low back or a general feeling of weekness. Standing straight, sitting and rising should be performed without pain. Sneezing and straining should not aggravate or cause you to have acute symptoms.

Stage 3—Chronic Rehabilitative Stage

You will reach this level when most of the symptoms of the acute and subacute stage have subsided, or where maximum improvement in your condition has been obtained. Long-term strengthening of the low back is essential to maintain your progress.

The following exercises are designed for acute and chronic back pain. They may be used by individuals who want a preventive program to help protect themselves against future episodes of back pain. Always consult your doctor before you begin any exercise program, particularly if you have had back surgery or multiple episodes of previous back pain. Arthritis or some muscular conditions can be aggravated by certain exercises. There are many exercises to fit your specific needs. The following exercises require some flexion (forward bending) and extension (backward bending). They are designed to restore normal function and mobility to the spine as well as to reduce the severity of the pain.

Exercise can alter your pain by increasing or decreasing it, and/or by changing its location. For example, if exercising causes your pain to move towards the spine and away from areas where the pain was previously felt, that is usually a good indicator that the exercise program is correct for you. If, however, the exercise or activity causes the pain to move away from the spine and perhaps increase the pain in the leg or buttock region, this is an indication that the exercise may be incorrect or the wrong position for your particular problem. There may be an increase in pain during the initial phase of any exercise. This is common and should subside after the first or second session, or the exercise should be discontinued. Consult your doctor if pain persists.

CAUTION

No exercise program should be undertaken without the approval, instruction and monitoring of your doctor of chiropractic.

Exercise—Acute Pain Stage

Knee to Chest

SETS	REPETITIONS per SET

1.

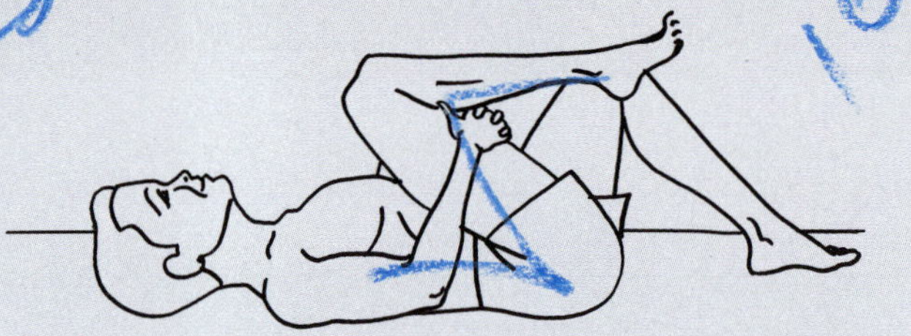

1. Lie flat on the floor in a relaxed position. Your left knee should be in a bent position with foot on floor. Bring your right knee toward your chest, clasping your hands behind the knee. Pull your right knee toward your chest firmly and hold for ten or twenty seconds and slowly relax. Repeat the same procedure with the opposite leg. Do as many sets or repetitions as recommended by your doctor.

Note: If back pain becomes worse when you bend backwards, these exercise positions are more likely to help. They are designed to move your body in positions which are not painful. If you experience pain, discontinue exercise and consult your doctor.

Bridging

2a.

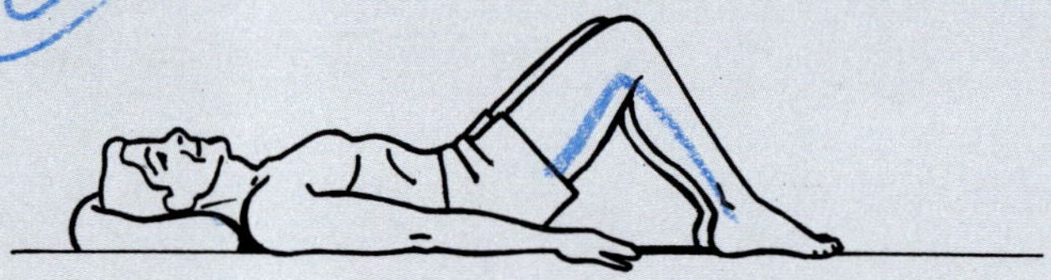

2a. To start the bridging exercise, lie on the floor with back flat, knees bent and feet flat on floor. Pillow under your head to prevent neck from arching back.

SETS	REPETITIONS per SET

2b.

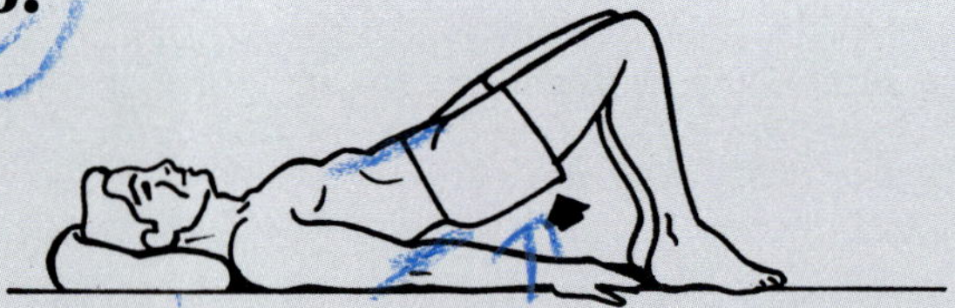

2b. Tighten the muscles of your lower abdomen and buttocks so as to flatten your low back. Slowly raise low back and buttocks from the floor and hold for ten to thirty seconds. Slowly relax. Do as many sets or repetitions as recommended by your doctor.

Pelvic Tilt

SETS	REPETITIONS per SET

3.

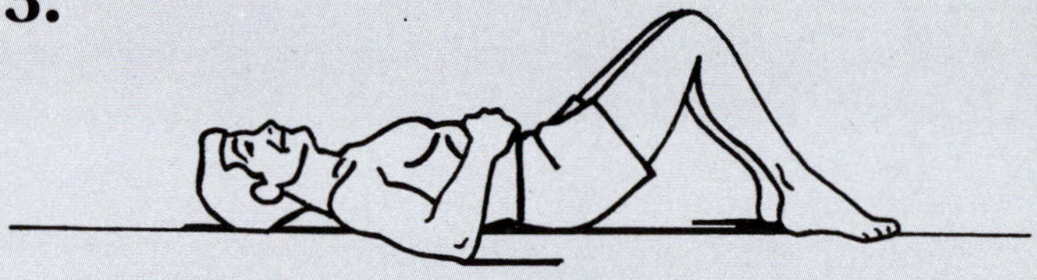

3. This is an important exercise in that it reduces stress on the lower back, especially when you are sitting or standing. You should lie on your back, knees bent, head comfortable with pillow. You may notice a space between your lower back and the surface of the floor. Squeeze your buttocks together, tighten abdominal muscles, and raise your buttocks until the small of your back is pressing flat against the surface of the floor. Hold for ten to twenty seconds and slowly relax. Do as many sets or repetitions as recommended by your doctor.

Extension Lying Prone

4a.

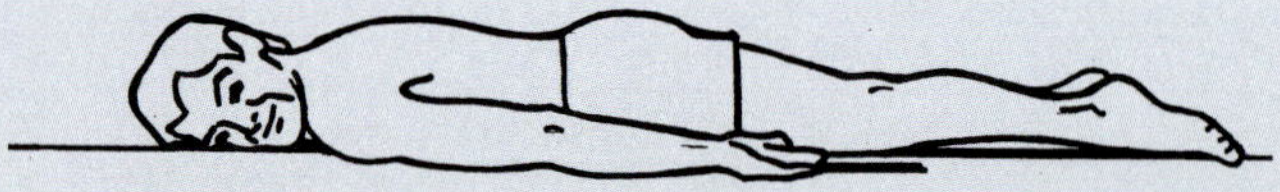

4a. Lie face down in a resting position. Relax and take a few deep breaths to release the tension in the lower back. Hold this position a few seconds until comfortable.

4b.

SETS	REPETITIONS per SET

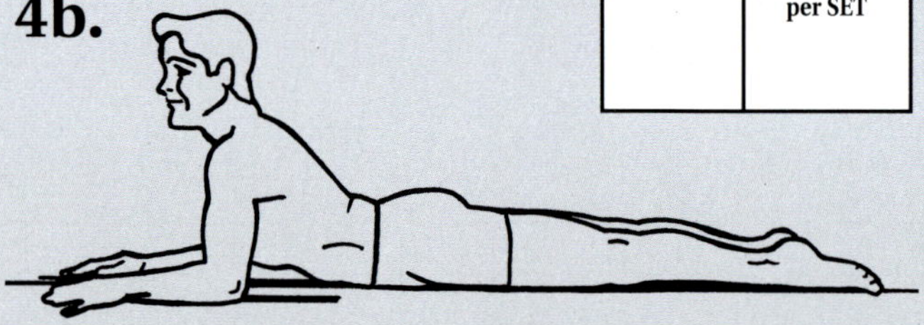

4b. Slide your forearms forward until your elbows are perpendicular to the floor. Then slowly raise your upper body as far as you can without increasing your pain. Hold this position for at least 30 seconds. This exercise should be performed only as many times as indicated by your doctor.

Note: This exercise is designed to stretch abdomen and hip flexors.

Note: Extension exercises are usually more helpful if back pain is worse when you sit or bend forward. Many people find their pain is relieved by performing extension exercises. Often times exercise programs are trial and error until you find the correct combination.

Exercise—Subacute/Recovery Stage

These exercises are to be performed in addition to those suggested during the acute stage of your condition.

Double Knee to Chest

SETS	REPETITIONS per SET

5.

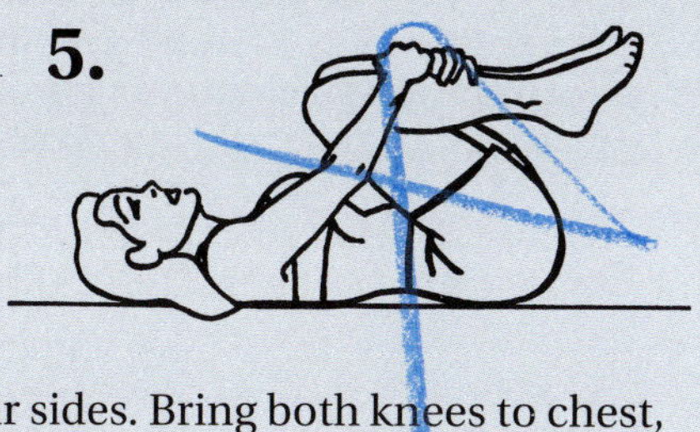

5. Lie on the floor with your knees bent, feet on the floor and arms at your sides. Bring both knees to chest, clasping hands around the knees and pulling firmly towards your chest. Hold for three to five seconds. Slowly relax. Do as many sets or repetitions as recommended by your doctor.

Hamstring Stretch

SETS	REPETITIONS per SET

6.

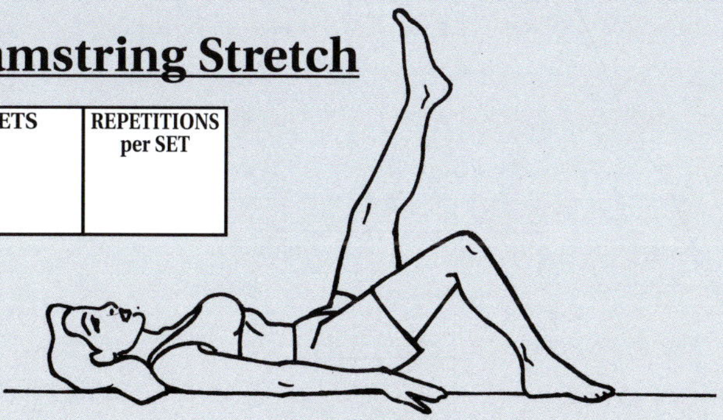

6. Lie on your back, your knees bent with feet flat on the floor, arms at your sides, palms down. Raise your left leg up as far as is comfortable without over-stretching muscles behind the leg. Return left leg to starting position and repeat five times. Repeat exercise with right leg. Do as many sets or repetitions as recommended by your doctor.

Note: Be certain to contract the abdominal muscles while keeping the lower back in contact with the floor. This exercise will help the muscles behind your thighs to be more flexible.

Hip Rotator Exercise

SETS	REPETITIONS per SET

7.

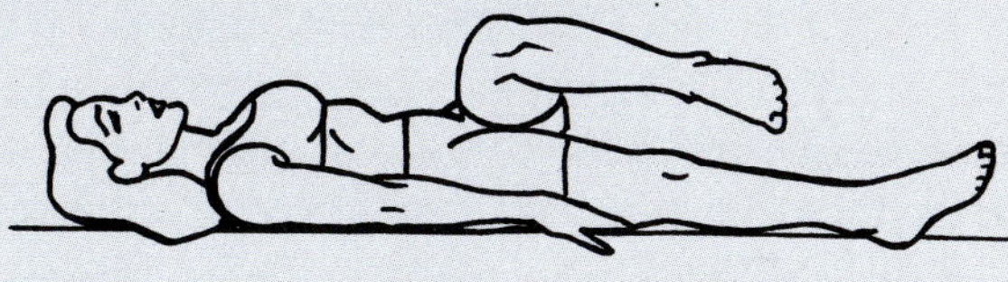

7. Lie flat on your back, arms at your sides, palms down. Slowly raise one leg, bringing the raised leg toward the opposite side of the body until you feel the stretch. Return to neutral position. Repeat with opposite leg. Do as many sets or repetitions as recommended by your doctor.

Note: Never stretch to the point of pain. If any exercise causes pain in your buttocks; pain, tingling or numbness in your legs, do not continue the exercise.

Calf Stretch

8.

SETS	REPETITIONS per SET

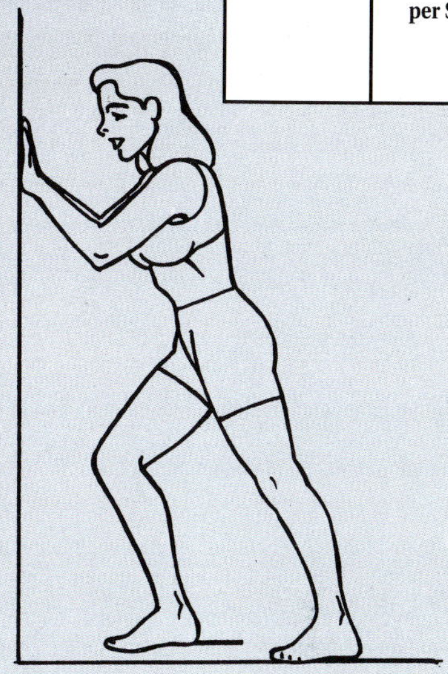

8. Standing with hands against wall, left foot approximately eighteen inches behind right foot, keeping heel flat on the floor and left knee straight, slowly bend forward until you feel the stretch behind the calf. Hold for three to five seconds, release the tension and repeat three to five times. Repeat with the opposite leg. This exercise is designed to release tension behind calf.

Abdominal Toning Exercise

SETS	REPETITIONS per SET

9.

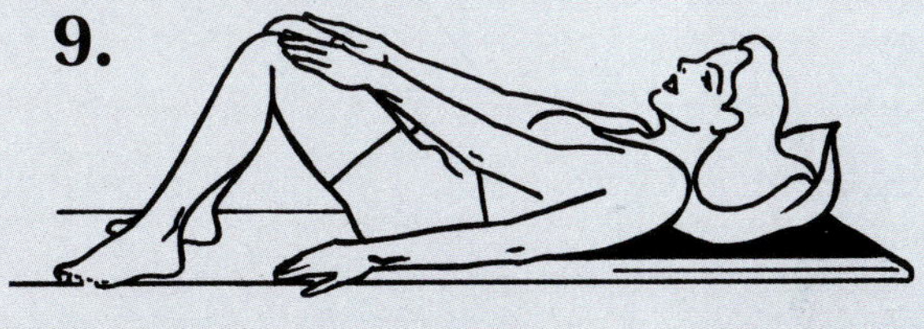

9. Lie with knees bent. Arms extended. Raise your head and shoulders from the floor until your hands touch your knees. Hold for three seconds, slowly uncurl and relax. Do as many sets or repetitions as recommended by your doctor.

Abdominal Toning Exercise

10.

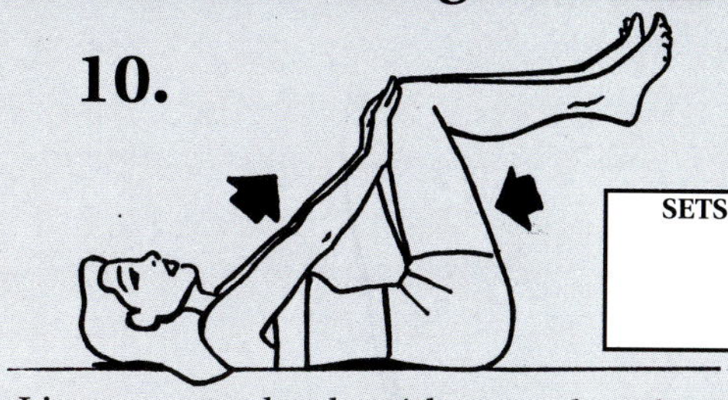

SETS	REPETITIONS per SET

10. Lie on your back with your hands against your thighs. Place a pillow under the small of your back to take up the space. Raise your legs so that your thighs will be perpendicular to the floor. It may be more comfortable to place an ottoman under your knees when doing this exercise. Push against your thighs with your hands while at the same time resisting with your thighs. Do this for ten to thirty seconds. Slowly relax. Do as many sets or repetitions as recommended by your doctor.

Exercise—Chronic/Rehabilitative Stage

Before you begin any exercise program, be certain that you begin by trying the movements slowly and carefully. Allow the muscles to loosen up. Mild heat or a hot tub soak for five to ten minutes prior to beginning the exercises may help to relax tight muscles.

Hamstring Stretch

11. Lie on your back, with both knees bent, feet flat on the floor. Bring one knee to the chest, then straighten it to the vertical position, pointing the toe upward as far as possible. Bend knee back to chest and return to original position. Repeat with opposite leg. Do as many sets or repetitions as recommended by your doctor.

11.

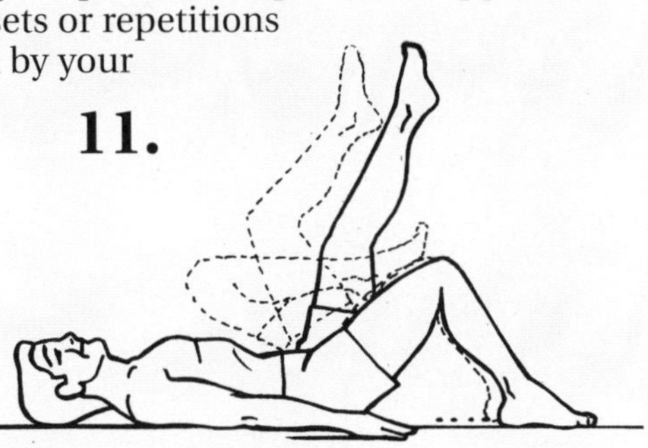

SETS	REPETITIONS per SET

Hamstring Stretch Sitting

12. Sit sideways on couch, stretch out right leg flat and put left foot on floor. Put left hand on left knee and reach forward with your right hand for the toes of the right foot. Reach as far forward as you can without discomfort. Feel the stretch behind the right leg, hold for three to five seconds and lean back to release the tension. Repeat with same leg five times, then change position and repeat with opposite leg.

SETS	REPETITIONS per SET

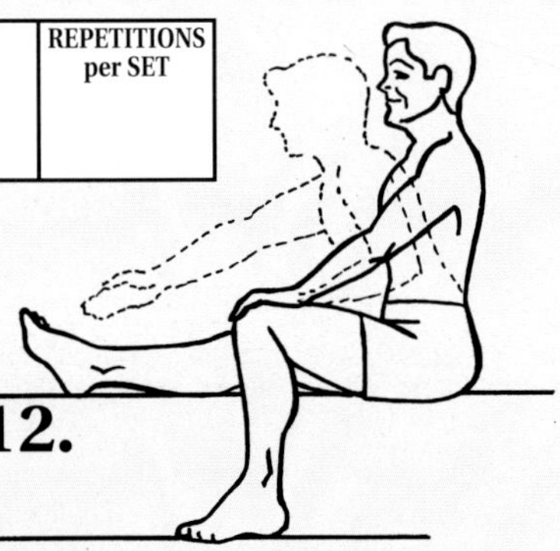

12.

Note: Be certain to maintain the lumbar curve when doing this exercise. Bend at the waist, not at the neck and shoulders.

13.

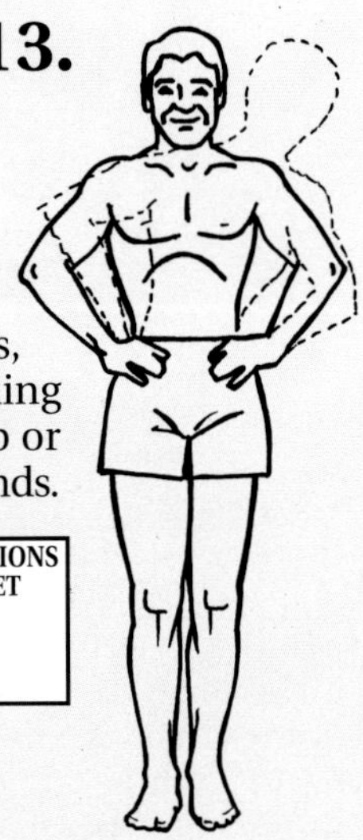

Side Stretching

13. Standing with hands on hips, bend slowly to one side, bending only at the waist. Do not flex hip or knee. Hold for three to five seconds. Return to neutral position and repeat to opposite side. Do as many sets or repetitions as recommended by your doctor.

SETS	REPETITIONS per SET

Abdominal Toning Exercise

14. Lie on back, knees bent, feet flat on floor, do not put hands behind head. It may be helpful to have someone hold your feet for support. Sit up to one quarter of a sitting position and hold for three to five seconds. Slowly relax. Do as many sets or repetitions as recommended by your doctor.

SETS	REPETITIONS per SET

14.

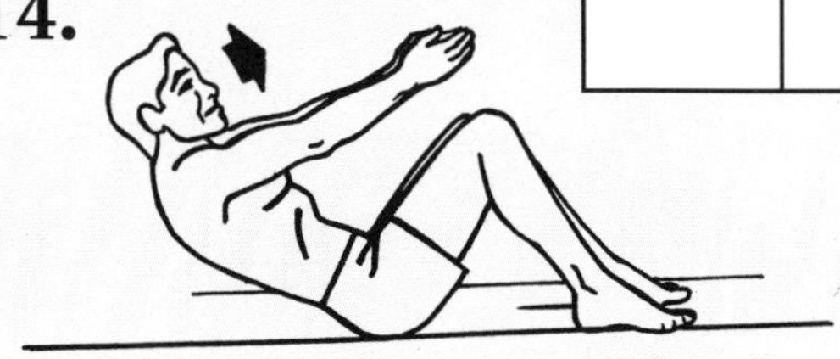

Prone Extension Exercise

15.

SETS	REPETITIONS per SET

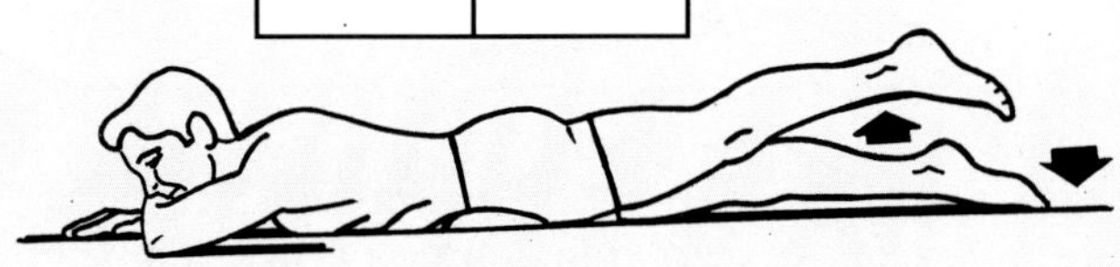

15. Lie face down on floor with large pillow under the hips and lower part of the abdomen. Lift one leg from the floor keeping the leg straight, hold for three to five seconds and slowly relax. Repeat using the other leg. Do as many sets or repetitions as recommended by your doctor.

Back Extension

SETS	REPETITIONS per SET

16.

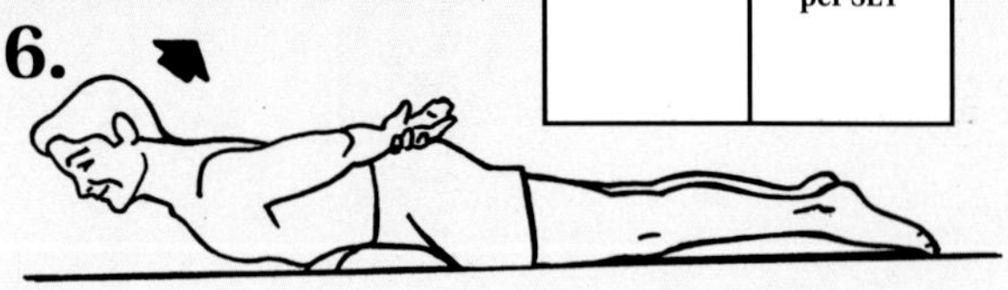

16. Lie face down on the floor with a pillow under your hips and the lower part of your abdomen. Place your hands behind your hips and lift your head and shoulders from the floor. You must be cautious not to raise your body high enough to cause pain in your lower back. Hold for three to five seconds, slowly relax and resume resting position. Do as many sets or repetitions as recommended by your doctor.

Side Lying Leg Lifts

SETS	REPETITIONS per SET

17.

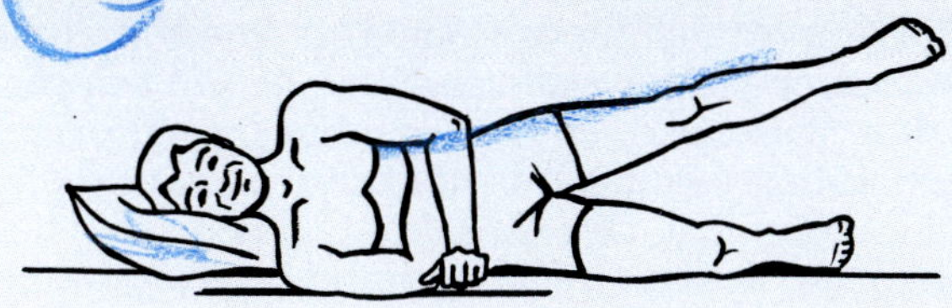

17. Lie on your right side, raise left leg to as near a vertical position as possible, repeat five times. Lie on left side and repeat the exercise raising right leg. Do as many sets or repetitions as recommended by your doctor.

Back Strength Training

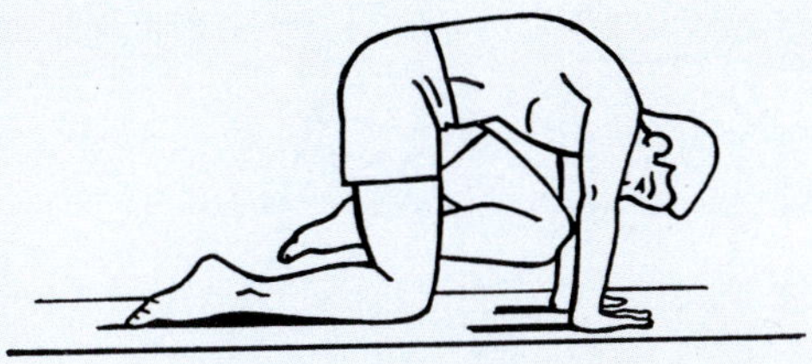

SETS	REPETITIONS per SET

18.

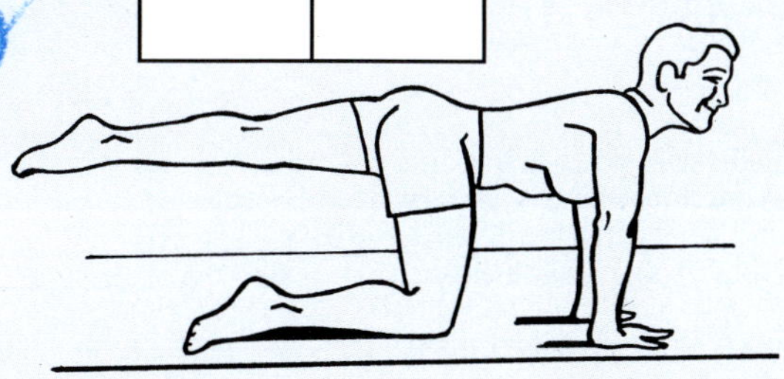

18. On hands and knees, draw one knee toward chest, flexing trunk and neck at same time. Then swing leg back to the outstretched position, extending neck and back at the same time. Do not extend the raised leg higher then level with floor. Repeat with other leg. Do as many sets or repetitions as recommended by your doctor.

tight abdomen + buttocks + keep tight in cat curl

Cat Curl Exercise

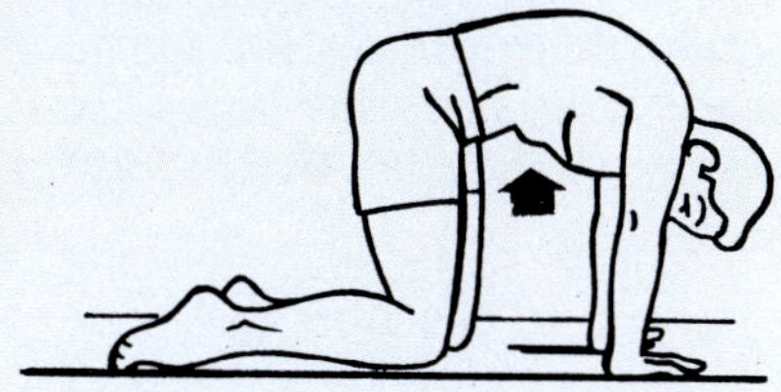

SETS	REPETITIONS per SET

19.

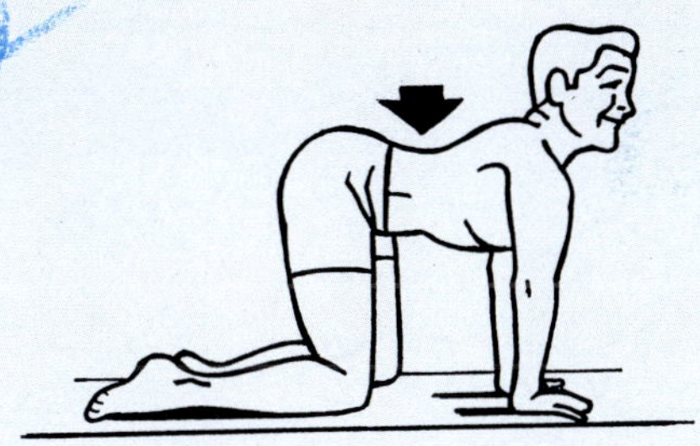

19. Assume a kneeling position, resting on your hands and knees. Arch your back like a cat, drop your head at the same time. Then, as illustrated reverse the arch by bringing up your head and forming a "U" with your spine. Do as many sets or repetitions as recommended by your doctor.

Oblique Abdominal Curl

20.

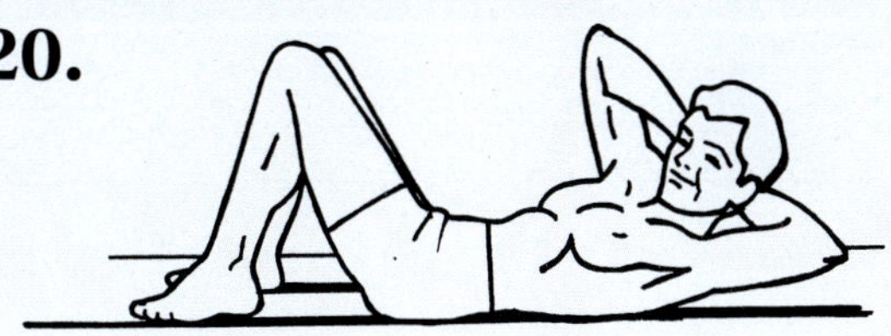

SETS	REPETITIONS per SET

20. Lie on back, knees bent, feet flat on the floor, hands behind neck. Begin to rotate your torso from a flat position with your right elbow reaching to the left side as illustrated. Hold for three to five seconds and then slowly relax. Turn in the opposite direction and repeat the exercise. Slowly relax back to the neutral position. Do as many sets or repetitions as recommended by your doctor.

Lying Extension Exercises

21. Lie face down with hands positioned to lift your body (21a.). Straighten your elbows and push the top half of your body as far as you can without experiencing pain (21b.). Maintain this position for a few seconds and then lower yourself to the floor as in the starting position. Each time you attempt to do this exercise try to raise your upper body a bit higher so your back is extended as far as you can comfortably go (21c.). Try to maintain this position for ten to twenty seconds and notice if the pain is reduced. Do as many sets or repetitions as recommended by your doctor.

21a.

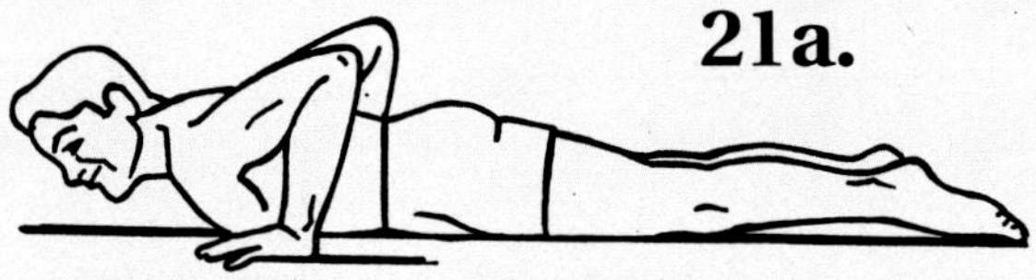

21b.

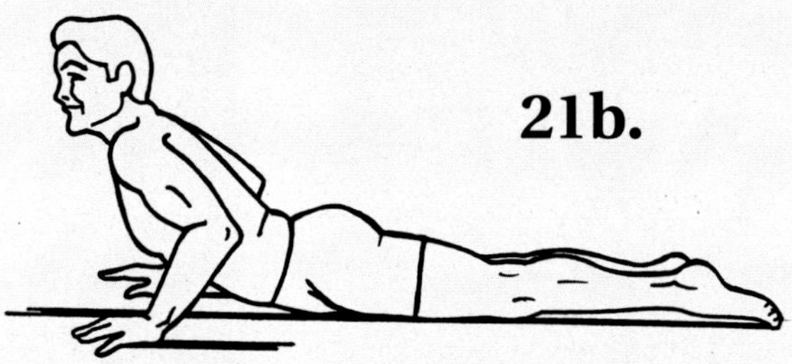

21c.

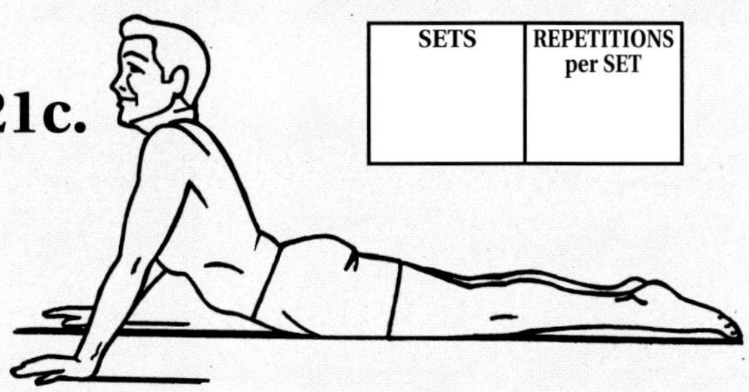

SETS	REPETITIONS per SET

Standing Extension Exercise

22. Stand with feet slightly apart. Place your hands in the small of your back with your fingers resting comfortably on your hips. Bend your body backward at the waist as far as you can, using your hands to help you extend (22.). Hold for five seconds and return slowly to the starting position. It is important that you keep your knees straight. Each time you repeat this exercise, try to bend backward a little further. This will often help in relieving acute back pain. The standing extension is not quite as effective as the Lying Extension Exercise (21.), but can be used when you are unable to lie down. The standing extension exercise is excellent to do when you have been in a forward position, as a stretching exercise. Do as many set or repetitions as recommended by your doctor.

SETS	REPETITIONS per SET

22.

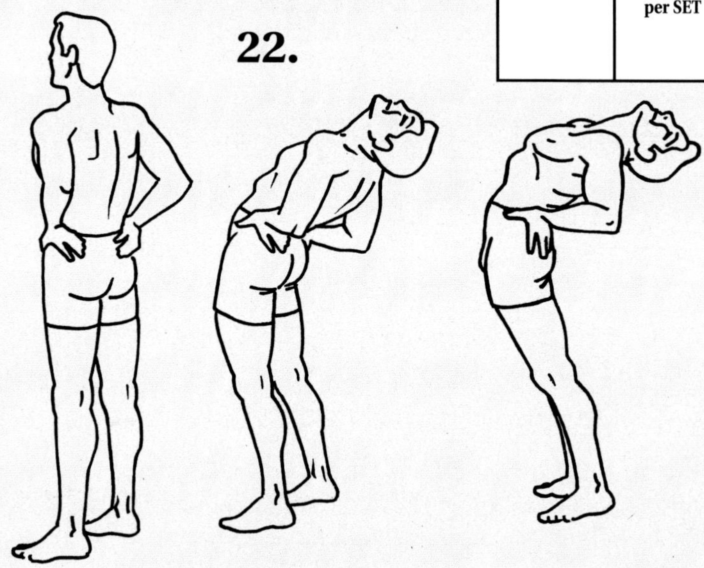

23a.Stand with your back against a wall, and position your feet approximately one foot away from the wall, and slightly apart. Relax your shoulders.

23b. Slowly sink straight down to about a 45 degree angle and hold for approximately twenty seconds. Slowly slide back up the wall. Do as many sets or repetitions as recommended by your doctor.

This exercise is designed to strengthen your muscles which should be used when lifting: the hamstring, buttock, and quadriceps muscles. It will help you strengthen this muscle group, which should be used, instead of your lower back muscles, when you are lifting heavy objects.

SETS	REPETITIONS per SET

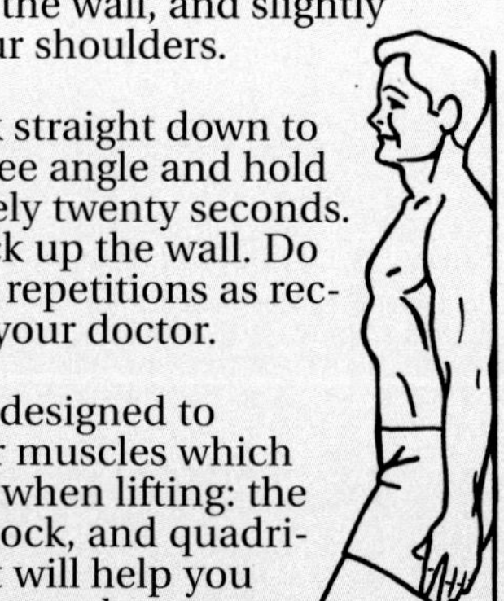

23a.

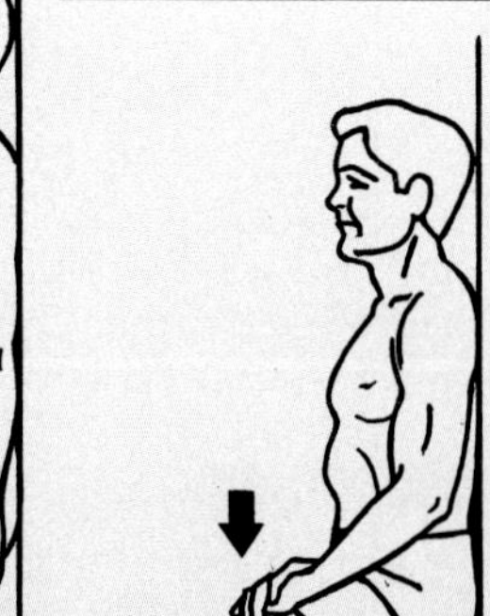

23b.

Exercises To Stretch And Restore Range Of Motion To The Neck

Note: Do not forcefully move your head when doing any of these movements. If you experience pain, dizziness, loss of balance or similar symptoms, stop the movement or exercise immediately. Contact your doctor for further advice.

The following is a group of mobilizing and stretching exercises designed to increase the range of motion in your cervical spine (neck). As you gain mobility in your neck, you should notice greater movement and less stiffness. Do not use any additional weights or devices when doing these exercises. Application of moist heat before you start may aid in your ability to perform these movements.

Flexion - Extension

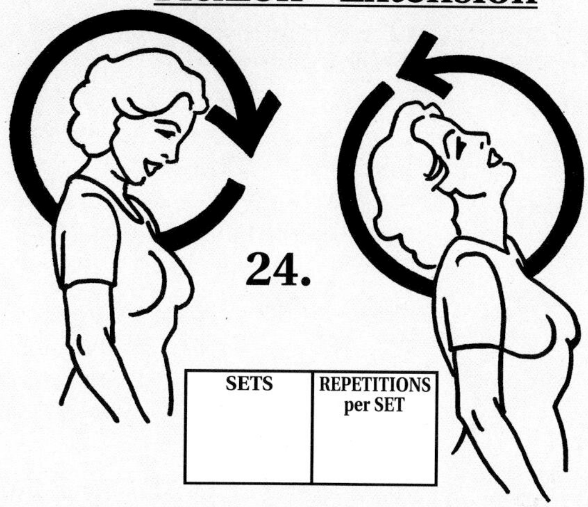

24.

SETS	REPETITIONS per SET

24. Tuck your chin. Gently bend the head forward, attempting to touch your chin to your chest. Gently bend your head backwards to its limit. Do as many sets or repetitions as recommended by your doctor.

Side Bending

SETS	REPETITIONS per SET

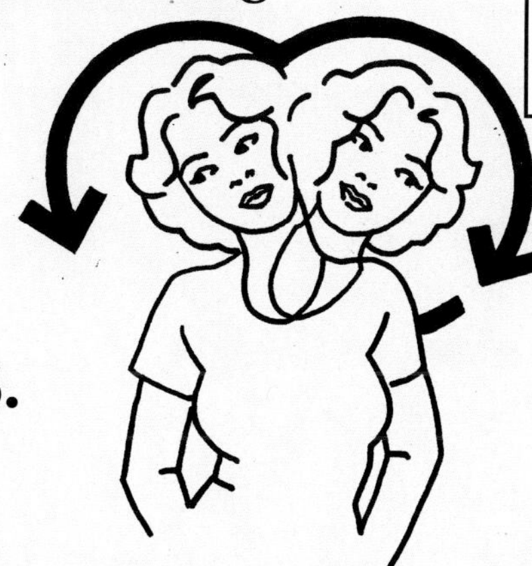

25.

25. Bend the head to the right as far as possible, attempting to touch your ear to your right shoulder. Do not rotate your head when doing this exercise. Bend the head to the left and repeat the exercise. Do as many sets or repetitions as recommended by your doctor.

Neck Rotation

SETS	REPETITIONS per SET

26.

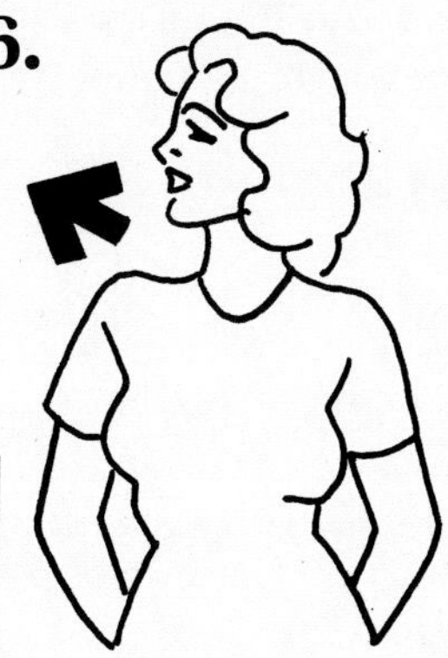

26. Turn head to the right as far as possible, attempting to bring chin over shoulder. Do not elevate shoulder. Hold three to five seconds.Repeat on the opposite side. Do as many sets or repetitions as recommended by your doctor.

Lateral Bending

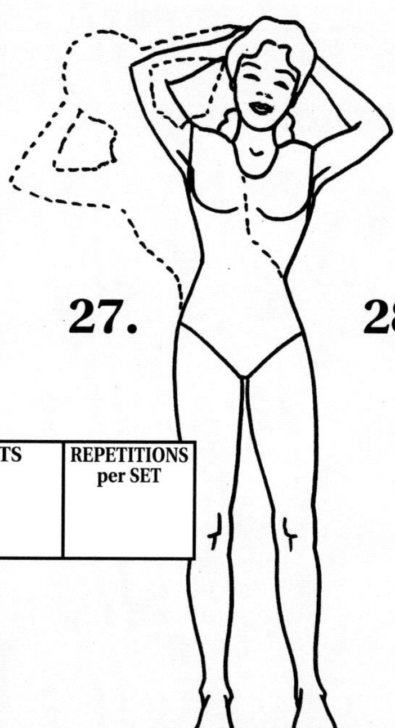

27.

SETS	REPETITIONS per SET

Chest Stretch

SETS	REPETITIONS per SET

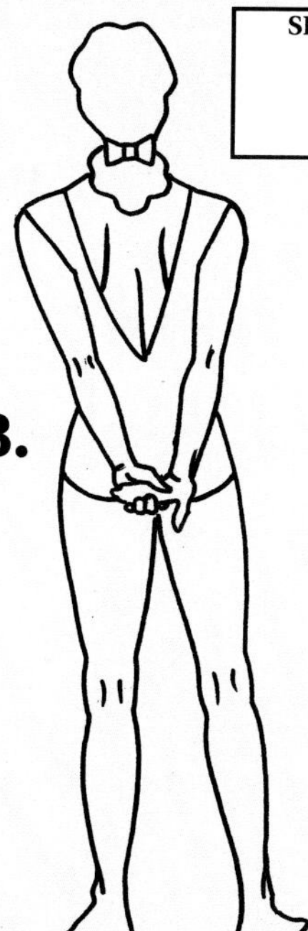

28.

27. Standing with feet apart, place hands behind head. Bend from side to side, bending only with the upper back. Do not bend the waist or hips. Attempt to reach the upper elbow to the ceiling. Hold each movement for three to five seconds. Alternate sides. Do as many sets or repetitions as recommended by your doctor.

28. Standing with feet apart, clasping hands behind the back, pull downward toward the floor with hands. Take a deep breath, stand on toes and look at the ceiling while exerting the downward pull. Hold for three to five seconds, then exhale slowly and relax. Do as many sets or repetitions as recommended by your doctor.

Exercises To Strengthen The Neck

The following is a group of isometric exercises designed to strengthen your neck muscles. If any of these exercises causes pain, dizziness, loss of balance, or other similar symptoms, stop the exercise immediately and contact your doctor. Do not use any additional weights or devices when doing these neck exercises. An application of moist heat before you begin your exercise program will often lessen the soreness caused by performing the exercises.

Flexion Isometric

29.

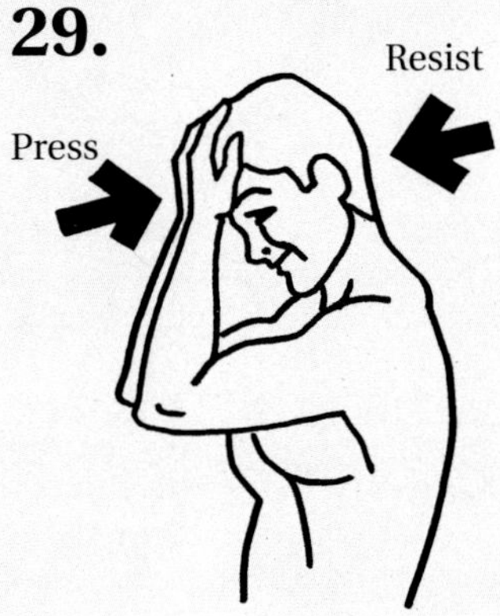

29. Press Your palms against your forehead and push against each other, resisting motion. Hold for 5 seconds, slowly relax. Do exercise three times per set. Do as many sets or repetitions as recommended by your doctor.

SETS	REPETITIONS per SET

Lateral Isometric

30.

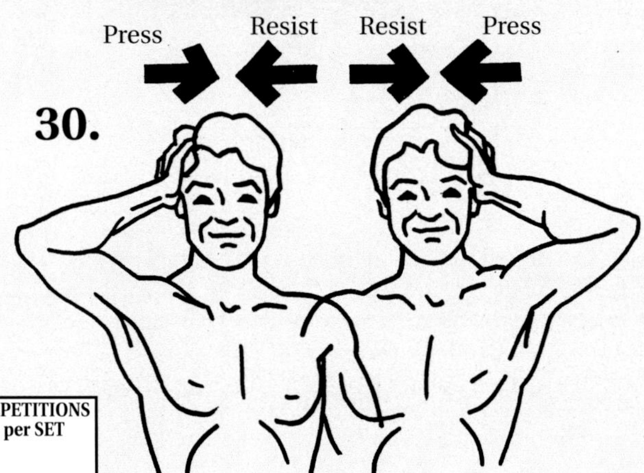

30. Place your hand against the side of your head. Attempt to bring your ear to your shoulder, resisting motion. Repeat the exercise on the opposite side. Hold for 5 seconds, slowly relax. Do as many sets or repetitions as recommended by your doctor.

SETS	REPETITIONS per SET

Extension Isometric

SETS	REPETITIONS per SET

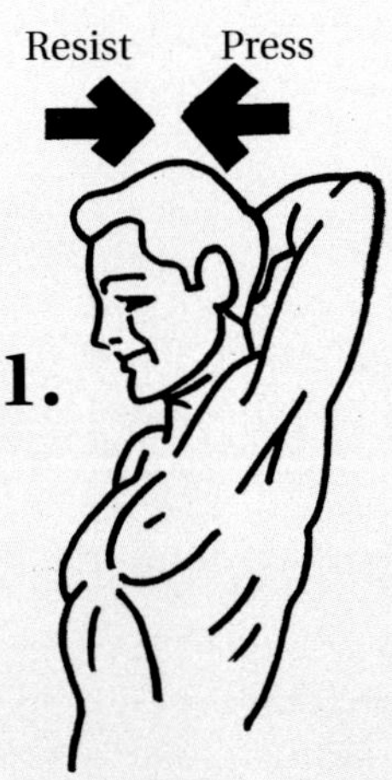

31.

31. Cup both hands against the back of your head. Try to push your head back, resisting motion. Hold for 5 seconds, slowly relax. Do as many sets or repetitions as recommended by your doctor.

Rotation Isometric

32.

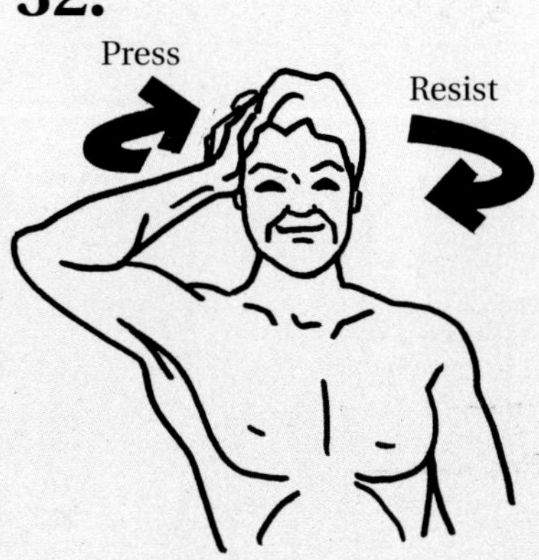

SETS	REPETITIONS per SET

32. Place your right hand against your right temple. Attempt to turn your chin to your right shoulder, resisting motion. Repeat exercise on opposite side. Hold for 5 seconds, slowly relax. Do as many sets or repetitions as recommended by your doctor.

References

1. Palmer DD. Textbook of Science, Art and Philosophy of Chiropractic. Portland, OR: Portland Printing House, 1910.
2. Biron WA, Wells BF, Houser RH. Chiropractic Principles and Technic, Chicago, IL: National College of Chiropractic, 1939
3. Kunert W. Functional disorders of internal organs due to vertebral lesions. Ciba Symposium 1965; 13: 85-96.
4. Lewit K. The contribution of clinical observation to neurobiological mechanisms in manipulative therapy. In Korr, IM. The Neurobiologic Mechanisms in Manipulative Therapy. New York, NY: Plenum Press, 1978, pp. 3-25.
5. Rychikova E. Vertebrogenic disorders in internal affections, their importance in therapy. In Lewit K, Gutzmann G, eds. Rehabilitacia, Proceedings of the 10th Congress, International Federation of Manipulative Medicine, Prague, CZECH REPUBLIC, 1975; suppl. 10-11: 94-95.
6. Harper WD. Anything Can Cause Anything. Houston, TX: Texas Chiropractic College, 1974.
7. Scofield AG. Chiropractic: The Science of Specific Spinal Adjusting. Wellingborough, Northamptonshire, UNITED KINGDOM: Thorsons Publishers Limited Denington Estate, 1968.
8. Leach RA. The Chiropractic Theories-A Synopsis of Scientific Research. Baltimore, MD: Williams and Wilkins, 1986.
9. Waddell G. A new clinical model for the treatment of back pain. Spine 1987; 12(7): 632-644.
10. Benson H, Greenwood MM, Klemchuk H. The relaxation response: Psychophysiologic aspects and clinical applications. International Journal of Psychiatry and Medicine 1975; 6(1): 87-98.
11. Ader R, Cohen H, Felten D. Psychoneuroimmunology: Interactions between the nervous system and the immune system. Lancet 1995; 345: 99-103.
12. Johnson E, Kamilars T, Chrousos G, Gold P. Mechanisms of stress: A dynamic overview of hormonal and behavioral homeostasis. Neuroscientific and Biobehavioral Review 1992; 16: 115-130.
13. Morgan LG. Psychoneuroimmunology, the placebo effect and chiropractic. Journal of Manipulative and Physiological Therapeutics 1998; 21(7): 484-491.
14. Schmorl G, Jonghans H. The Human Spine in Health and Disease. New York, NY: Grune & Stratton, 1971.
15. Verhoef MJ, Page SA, Waddell G. The Chiropractic Outcome Study: Pain, functional ability and satisfaction with care. Journal of Manipulative and Physiological Therapeutics 1997; 20(4): 235-240.
16. Vernon H, Mior S. The neck disability index: A study of reliability and validity. Journal of Manipulative and Physiological Therapeutics 1991; 14(7): 409-415.
17. Haldeman S. Principles and Practice of Chiropractic. Norwalk, CT: Appleton & Lang, 1992.
18. Korr IM. The neural basis of the osteopathic lesion. Journal of the American Osteopathic Association 1947; 47: 191-198.
19. Budgell B. The reflex effects of subluxation: The autonomic nervous system. Symposium Proceedings of the World Federation of Chiropractic, Auckland, NEW ZEALAND, May 18-21, 1999, pp. 20-25.
20. Breen AC. Chiropractors and the treatment of back pain. Rheumatology and Rehabilitation 1977; 16(1): 46-53.
21. Kokjohn K, Schmid DM, Triano JJ, Brennan PC. The effect of spinal manipulation on pain and prostaglandin levels in women with primary dysmenorrhea. Journal of Manipulative and Physiological Therapeutics 1992; 15(5): 279-285.
22. Walsh MJ, Chandraraj S, Polus BI. The efficacy of chiropractic therapy on premenstrual syndrome: A case series study. Chiropractic Journal of Australia 1994; 24(4): 122-126.
23. Klougart N, Nilsson N, Jacobsen J. Infantile colic treated by chiropractors: A prospective study of 316 cases. Journal of Manipulative and Physiological Therapeutics 1989; 12(4): 281-288.
24. Reed WR, Beavers S, Reddy SK, Kern G. Chiropractic management of primary nocturnal enuresis. Journal of Manipulative and Physiological Therapeutics 1994; 17(9): 596-600.
25. Yates RG, Lamping DL, Abram NL, Wright C. Effects of chiropractic treatment on blood pressure and anxiety: A randomized, controlled trial. Journal of Manipulative and Physiological Therapeutics 1989; 11(6): 484-488.
26. Egli AB. Spine and heart: Vertebrogenous cardiac syndromes. Annals of the Swiss Chiropractic Association 1965; 4: 95-105.
27. Tran TA, Kirby JD. The effects of upper cervical adjustments on the normal physiology of the heart. Journal of the American Chiropractic Association 1977; 14: s59-s62.
28. Gamble A. Alternative medical approaches to the treatment of asthma. Alternative and Complementary Therapies in Health and Medicine 1995; 1(2): 61-66.
29. Jamison JR, McEwen AP, Thomas SJ. Chiropractic adjustment in the management of visceral conditions: A critical appraisal. Journal of Manipulative and Physiological Therapeutics 1992; 15(3): 171-180.
30. Jamison JR. Preventive chiropractic and the chiropractic management of visceral conditions. Chiropractic Journal of Australia 1991; 21(3):95-101.
31. Pikalov AA, Kharin VV. Use of spinal manipulative therapy in the treatment of duodenal ulcer: A pilot study. Journal of Manipulative and Physiological Therapeutics 1994; 17(5): 310-313.
32. Wagner T, Owen J, Malone E, Mann K. Irritable bowel syndrome and spinal manipulation: A case report.Chiropractic Technique 1995; 7(4): 139-140.
33. Wells BF, Janse JJ. Chiropractic Practice, vol. 2. Lombard, IL: National College of Chiropractic, 1943.
34. Stoddard A. Manual of Osteopathic Technic. Hagerstown, MD: Harper and Row, 1969.
35. Bourdillon JF, Day EA. Spinal Manipulation, 4th edition. New York, NY: Appleton & Lange, 1987.
36. Weiant CW, Goldschmidt S. Medicine and Chiropractic. Lombard, IL: National College of Chiropractic, 1975.
37. Williams PL. Grays Anatomy, edition 38. New York, NY: Churchill Livingstone, 1995, p. 1293.
38. Merkin JJ, Sportelli L. The effects of two new compensating filters on patient exposure in chiropractic full spine radiography: A technical report. Journal of Manipulative and Physiological Therapeutics 1982; 5(1): 25-29.
39. Van Schaik JPJ, Verbiest H, Van Schaik FDJ. Isolated spinous process deviations. A pitfall in the interpretation of the lumbar spine. Spine 1989; 14(9): 970-976.
40. Taylor JAM. The role of radiography in evaluating subluxation. In Gatterman M [ed.], Foundations of Chiropractic Subluxation. St. Louis, MO: Mosby-Year Book, 1995, pp. 68-86.
41. Gillet H. Vertebral fixations, an introduction to movement palpation. Annals of the Swiss Chiropractic Association 1960: 1: 30.
42. Schafer RC, Faye LJ. Motion Palpation and Chiropractic Technique: Principles of Dynamic Chiropractic. Huntington Beach, CA: Motion Palpation Institute, 1991.
43. Grecco M. Chiropractic Technic Illustrated. New York, NY: Harl Publishing Co., 1953.
44. Levine M. The Structural Approach to Chiropractic. New York, NY: Comet Press, 1964.
45. Bergmann T, Peterson D, Lawrence D. Chiropractic Technique: Principles and Procedures. New York, NY: Churchill Livingstone, 1993.
46. Plaugher G, Cremata EE, Phillips RB. A retrospective consecutive case analysis of pretreatment and comparative static radiological parameters following chiropractic adjustments. Journal of Manipulative and Physiological Therapeutics 1990; 13(9): 498-506.

47. Breen AC, Allen R, Morris A. Spine kinematics: A digital videofluoroscopic technique. Journal of Biomedical Engineering 1989; 11: 224-228.
48. Haas M, Panzer DM. Palpatory diagnosis of subluxation. In Gatterman M [ed]. Foundations of Chiropractic Subluxation. St. Louis, MO: Mosby-Year Book, 1995, pp. 56-67.
49. Schultz G, Phillips RB, Cooley J, Hall T, Hoyt T, Gendreaud D, Knudsen JT, Mitchell R, Taylor JAM. Diagnostic imaging of the spine in chiropractic practice: Recommendations for utilization. Chiropractic Journal of Australia 1992; 22(4): 141-152.
50. Shekelle PG, Markovich M, Louie R. Comparing the costs between provider types of episodes of back pain care. Spine 1995; 20(2): 221-227.
51. Carey TS, Garrett J, Jackman A, McLaughlin C, Fryer J, Smucker DR, North Carolina Back Pain Project. New England Journal of Medicine 1995; 333(14): 913-917.
52. Basmajian J. Therapeutic Exercise. Baltimore, MD: Williams & Wilkins, 1982.
53. Schafer RC. Applied Physiotherapy. Arlington, VA: Associated Chiropractic Academic Press, 1986.
54. Janse JJ. An Anthology, Principles and Practice of Chiropractic. Lombard, IL: National College of Chiropractic, 1976.
55. Albanese, A. Bone Loss: Causes, Detection, and Therapy. New York, NY: Alan R. Liss Co., 1977.
56. Select Committee on Nutrition and Human Needs, U.S. Senate, Dietary Goals for United States, Washington, DC: U.S. Government Printing Office, 1977.
57. Walczak M. Nutrition Applied Personally, La Habra, CA: International College of Applied Nutrition, 1973.
58. Werbach M. Nutritional Influences on Illness. Tarzana, CA: Third Line Press, 1993.
59. Painter NS. Diverticular disease of the colon: The first of the Western diseases shown to be due to a deficiency of dietary fibre. South African Medical Journal 1982; 61(26): 1016-1020.
60. White A. III. Your Aching Back: A Doctor's Guide to Relief. New York, NY: Simon and Shuster, 1990.
61. The management of chronic pain in older persons: AGS Panel on Chronic Pain in Older Persons: American Geriatrics Society. Journal of the American Geriatric Society; 1998; 46(5): 635-651.
62. Cleave TL. The Saccharin Disease. New Canaan, CT: Keats Publishing Company, 1975.
63. The American Heart Association, An Eating Plan for Healthy Americans. New York, NY, 1986.
64. Noakes M, Clifton PM. Oil blends containing partially hydrogenated or interesterified fats: Differential effects on plasma lipids. American Journal of Clinical Nutrition 1988; 68(2): 242-247.
65. Buckett et al. Refined Carbohydrate Foods and Disease. New York, NY: Academic Press, 1975
66. Morgan T. et al. Hypertension treated by salt restriction. Lancet 1978; 326; 227-230.
67. Stunkard A. Obesity. Philadelphia, PA: WB Saunders Co., 1980.
68. Select Committee on Nutrition and Human Needs, U.S. Senate, Diet Related to Killer Diseases, Washington, DC: U.S. Government Printing Office, 1977.
69. Schafer RC. Chiropractic Management of Sports and Recreational Injuries. Baltimore, MD: Williams & Wilkins, 1986.
70. Coggins W. Basic Technic: A System of Body Mechanics. Creve Coeur, MO: Elco Publishing Co., 1983.
71. Lantz CA, Chen J. The effect of chiropractic full spine adjustments on adolescent idiopathic scoliosis with curves less than 20 degrees. Proceedings of the International Conference on Spinal Manipulation. Bournemouth, U.K. Foundation for Chiropractic Education and Research, October 1996, pp. 30-32.
72. Froehle RM. Ear infection: A retrospective study examining improvement from chiropractic care and analyzing for influencing factors. Journal of Manipulative and Physiological Therapeutis 1996; 19(3): 169-177.
73. Fallon JM. The role of the chiropractic adjustment in the care and treatment of 332 children with otitis media. Journal of Clinical Chiropractic Pediatrics 1997; 2(2): 167-183.
74. Maigne R. Orthopedic Medicine: A New Approach to Vertebral Manipulations. Springfield, IL: Charles C. Thomas Publisher, 1979.
75. Rupert RL. A survey of practice patterns and the health promotion and prevention attitudes of U.S. chiropractors: Maintenance care. Journal of Manipulative and Physiological Therapeutics 1998; in press.
76. Rupert RL. Maintenance care: Health promotion services administered to U.S. chiropractic patients age 65 and older. Journal of Manipulative and Physiological Therapeutics 1998; in press.
77. Kirkaldy-Willis WH. Managing Low Back Pain. New York, NY: Churchill Livingstone, 1983.
78. Calliet R. Low Back Pain Syndrome, 4th edition. Philadelphia, PA: F.A. Davis, 1988.
79. Nwuga VCB. Relative therapeutic efficacy of vertebral manipulation and conventional treatment in back pain management. American Journal of Physical Medicine 1982; 61(6): 273-277.
80. Cox JM. Low Back Pain Mechanism: Diagnosis and Treatment. Baltimore, MD: Williams & Wilkins, 1985.
81. Buerger AA, Tobis JJ. Approaches to Validation of Manipulation Therapy. Springfield, IL: Charles C. Thomas Publishers, 1977.
82. Bigos S, Bowyer O, Braen G, et. al. Acute Low-Pain In Adults Clinical Practice Guideline No. 14, Agency for Health Care Policy and Research. Publication 95-0642. Rockville, MD: AHCPR, 1994.
83. Farfan HF. Mechanical Disorders of the Low Back. Philadelphia, PA: Lea & Feibiger, 1973.
84. Ciba Clinical Symposia, Low Back Pain. Summit, NJ: Ciba Pharmaceuticals, 1973.
85. McNab I. Backache. Baltimore, MD: Williams & Wilkins Co., 1977.
86. Ehni G. Cervical Arthrosis, Diseases of Cervical Motion Segments. Chicago, IL: Yearbook Medical Publishers, Inc., 1984.
87. Jackson R. The Cervical Syndrome, 4th edition. Springfield, IL: Charles C. Thomas Publishers, 1977.
88. Forman SM, Croft AC. Whiplash Injuries, The Cervical Acceleration/Deceleration Syndrome. Baltimore, MD: Williams & Wilkins, 1988.
89. Goff CW, Aldes JH, Alden JO. Traumatic Cervical Syndrome and Whiplash. Philadelphia, PA: JB Lippincott, 1967.
90. Kramer J. Intervertebral Disk Disease [Goldie IF, trans.]. Chicago, IL: Yearbook Medical Publishers, Inc., 1981.
91. Kisner C, Colby LA. Therapeutic Exercise: Foundations and Techniques, 3rd edition. Philadelphia, PA: F.A. Davis, 1996.
92. Leape LL. Unnecessary Surgery, Annual Review of Public Health, 1992; 13: 363-383
93. Shekelle PG et al. The Appropriateness of Spinal Manipulation for Low Back Pain: Project Overview and Literature Review, RAND, Santa Monica, CA: Monograph R-4025/1-CCR/FCER, 1991, p.3
94. Cramer, GD, Darby, SA, Basic and Clinical Anatomy of the Spine, Spinal Cord and ANA, St. Louis: Mosby, 1995.
95. Alternative Medicine, Inc. A multi-speciality IPA Highland Park Illinois, Richard L. Sarnet, M.D., personal correspondence, January 12, 2000.